Stikky™ Weight Management

Stikky™ Weight Management

IN ONE HOUR, LEARN TO BALANCE YOUR ENERGY INTAKE AND BURN RATE
TO CONTROL YOUR WEIGHT, OPTIMIZE YOUR HEALTH, AND LOOK GREAT.

LAURENCE HOLT BOOKS
New York

© 2004 Laurence Holt Books, Inc
www.stikky.com

303 Park Avenue South, #1030
New York, NY, 10010

First printing October 2003

Library of Congress Cataloging-in-Publication Data on file.

Cover design and illustrations by Kate Shannon.
Photography by Julian Lawson.

ISBN 1-932974-02-4

10 9 8 7 6 5 4 3 2

Printed in Canada

What this book is about

Stikky Weight Management uses a powerful learning method to teach anyone the skill of managing their weight, step-by-step.

Each step builds on what came before and reinforces it. That way, by the time you reach the end of the book, you will be confident in managing your weight for the rest of your life.

Still more exciting, the things you learn will serve as 'hooks' on which you can hang future knowledge.

This book also reveals the foods that are America's top sources of calories, saturated fat, and fiber, and the truth behind popular diets.

Stikky Weight Management has four parts:

- **Sequence One** explains why your weight increases or decreases and the *only two ways* you can affect it, helps you figure out your *target weight*, explains why a temporary diet has only a temporary effect, teaches you how to *gauge the calories* in foods, and how to *decipher nutrition labels*. *If possible, you should read this sequence in one sitting.*

- **Sequence Two** builds on what you have learned in Sequence One, explores the idea of *diet substitutions*, uncovers the latest findings on how much *exercise* you really need, and reveals the *three bad foods* and *four good ones*. *Ideally, you should leave a few days, but no more than a week, between completing Sequence One and starting Sequence Two.*

- **The Epilogue**, a special feature of Stikky books, brings together everything you have learned so far and reinforces it in some new and unfamiliar situations. *Again, you should leave a few days between completing Sequence Two and reading the Epilogue.*

- If, by the end of the book, you are eager to find out more, as we hope you will be, you will find dozens of things to explore in the **Next Steps** section.

You can skip to the Next Steps section at any time, of course, but the rest of the book only makes sense if read in order: Sequence One, Sequence Two, Epilogue.

How to read this book

Learning with *Stikky Weight Management* may be different from how you are used to learning.
Please read this page carefully.

First, read Sequence One which runs from the next page to the **Pause point** on page 121. That should take only 30 minutes (but don't worry if it takes longer).

We find people get more out of the book if they stop there and practice what they have learned for real. We'd like you to do the same.

Then, after a few days, read Sequence Two. If you are away from the book for more than a week, you may find it helpful to review some of Sequence One before starting Sequence Two.

Many people have read a lot about diet and formed deeply held views. But research on the topic is still unfolding, so we ask you to withhold judgement at least until you get to the end of this book. If you come across something that surprises you, keep in mind that everything here is based on research published in major scientific journals. Page-by-page references can be found at www.stikky.com.

To get the most from *Stikky Weight Management*:

- Relax and take your time
- Don't worry about taking notes
- Don't worry about memorizing anything
- Try to avoid being interrupted.

Most importantly, by turning this page you promise yourself that, when asked a question in the text, you will not flip ahead until you have tried to answer it.

(Flipping backwards to review pages you have already covered is fine.)

Keep this promise and what you learn will stick.

Sequence One

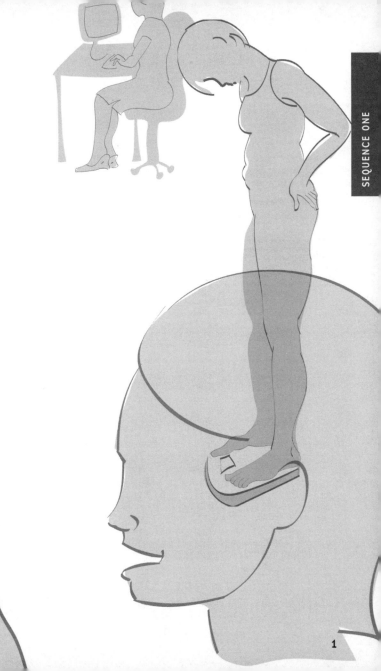

Your body is the most
remarkable machine you will
ever own.

It is also the most complex.

If you had an owner's handbook
for your body, it might read
something like this book.

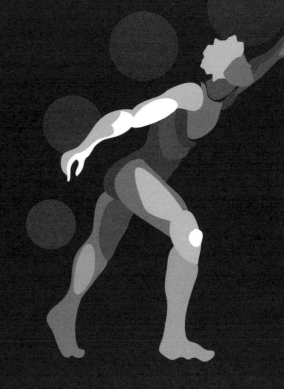

Here are the top six causes of serious breakdowns in American bodies—breakdowns that cause them to stop working for good.

Together, the top three account for 60% of all US deaths.

1	Heart diseases	29.6%
2	Cancers	23.0%
3	Cerebrovascular diseases (stroke)	7.0%
4	Chronic lower respiratory diseases (bronchitis, emphysema, asthma)	5.1%
5	Accidents	4.1%
6	Diabetes mellitus	2.9%

SOURCE: *Deaths: Leading Causes for 2000*, Centers for Disease Control and Prevention, www.cdc.gov/nchs

ONE

There are two simple things anyone can do to improve their body's chances of avoiding the top three risks (and many of the others).

The first is this: if you smoke, quit.

There is nothing in this book (or any other book, for that matter) that can offset the increased risk from smoking.

1	Heart diseases	29.6%
2	Cancers	23.0%
3	Cerebrovascular diseases (stroke)	7.0%
4	Chronic lower respiratory diseases (bronchitis, emphysema, asthma)	5.1%
5	Accidents	4.1%
6	Diabetes mellitus	2.9%

SOURCE: *Deaths: Leading Causes for 2000*, Centers for Disease Control and Prevention, www.cdc.gov/nchs

The second is: if you are overweight, lose it.

Being overweight is an epidemic in the US—two-thirds of Americans are overweight, and half of these are obese (twice the number from 20 years ago). The epidemic contributes to 300,000 American deaths each year.

Just one-third of Americans are at a healthy weight.

1	Heart diseases	29.6%
2	Cancers	23.0%
3	Cerebrovascular diseases (stroke)	7.0%
4	Chronic lower respiratory diseases (bronchitis, emphysema, asthma)	5.1%
5	Accidents	4.1%
6	Diabetes mellitus	2.9%

SOURCE: *Deaths: Leading Causes for 2000*, Centers for Disease Control and Prevention, www.cdc.gov/nchs

This table will help you find out if you are overweight and by how much, according to the official definition.

For instance, someone—male or female—who is 5 feet 8 inches tall should weigh less than 164 pounds. If they are 184 pounds, they are at least 20 pounds overweight.

If your height is:	You should weigh less than (pounds):
6 feet 6 inches	216
6 feet 5 inches	210
6 feet 4 inches	205
6 feet 3 inches	200
6 feet 2 inches	194
6 feet 1 inch	189
6 feet	184
5 feet 11 inches	179
5 feet 10 inches	174
5 feet 9 inches	169
5 feet 8 inches	164
5 feet 7 inches	159
5 feet 6 inches	154
5 feet 5 inches	150
5 feet 4 inches	145
5 feet 3 inches	141
5 feet 2 inches	136
5 feet 1 inch	132
5 feet	128
4 feet 11 inches	123
4 feet 10 inches	119

Being overweight increases your risk of dying early.

Overweight people are:
- Twice as likely to die from cardiovascular disease
- Three times as likely to have high blood pressure, and
- Four or more times as likely to develop diabetes.

A lower weight also means a lower risk of cancer, stroke and osteoarthritis. On average, being overweight shortens your life by three years.

If your height is:	You should weigh less than (pounds):
6 feet 6 inches	216
6 feet 5 inches	210
6 feet 4 inches	205
6 feet 3 inches	200
6 feet 2 inches	194
6 feet 1 inch	189
6 feet	184
5 feet 11 inches	179
5 feet 10 inches	174
5 feet 9 inches	169
5 feet 8 inches	164
5 feet 7 inches	159
5 feet 6 inches	154
5 feet 5 inches	150
5 feet 4 inches	145
5 feet 3 inches	141
5 feet 2 inches	136
5 feet 1 inch	132
5 feet	128
4 feet 11 inches	123
4 feet 10 inches	119

To allow a safety margin, experts recommend a good target weight would be several pounds less.

This target is shown in the column farthest right. (You may be surprised that the targets are the same for men and women —but that is the finding from detailed medical research).

If your height is:	You should weigh less than (pounds):	And a good target weight is:
6 feet 6 inches	216	190
6 feet 5 inches	210	186
6 feet 4 inches	205	181
6 feet 3 inches	200	176
6 feet 2 inches	194	171
6 feet 1 inch	189	167
6 feet	184	162
5 feet 11 inches	179	158
5 feet 10 inches	174	153
5 feet 9 inches	169	149
5 feet 8 inches	164	145
5 feet 7 inches	159	140
5 feet 6 inches	154	136
5 feet 5 inches	150	132
5 feet 4 inches	145	128
5 feet 3 inches	141	124
5 feet 2 inches	136	120
5 feet 1 inch	132	116
5 feet	128	113
4 feet 11 inches	123	109
4 feet 10 inches	119	105

Use this table to figure out your own target weight.

Make a note of the number, we'll need it later. Don't worry if it is very different from your current weight—given enough time, and the simple insights we are going to look at, you can achieve any weight you choose.

If your height is:	You should weigh less than (pounds):	And a good target weight is:
6 feet 6 inches	216	190
6 feet 5 inches	210	186
6 feet 4 inches	205	181
6 feet 3 inches	200	176
6 feet 2 inches	194	171
6 feet 1 inch	189	167
6 feet	184	162
5 feet 11 inches	179	158
5 feet 10 inches	174	153
5 feet 9 inches	169	149
5 feet 8 inches	164	145
5 feet 7 inches	159	140
5 feet 6 inches	154	136
5 feet 5 inches	150	132
5 feet 4 inches	145	128
5 feet 3 inches	141	124
5 feet 2 inches	136	120
5 feet 1 inch	132	116
5 feet	128	113
4 feet 11 inches	123	109
4 feet 10 inches	119	105

As well as the significant health benefits we already mentioned, people who reach their target weight report:

- Sleeping better
- Having more energy
- Feeling better about their appearance
- Gaining confidence.

Is there anything you could do or buy that provides as much benefit?

If your height is:	You should weigh less than (pounds):	And a good target weight is:
6 feet 6 inches	216	190
6 feet 5 inches	210	186
6 feet 4 inches	205	181
6 feet 3 inches	200	176
6 feet 2 inches	194	171
6 feet 1 inch	189	167
6 feet	184	162
5 feet 11 inches	179	158
5 feet 10 inches	174	153
5 feet 9 inches	169	149
5 feet 8 inches	164	145
5 feet 7 inches	159	140
5 feet 6 inches	154	136
5 feet 5 inches	150	132
5 feet 4 inches	145	128
5 feet 3 inches	141	124
5 feet 2 inches	136	120
5 feet 1 inch	132	116
5 feet	128	113
4 feet 11 inches	123	109
4 feet 10 inches	119	105

When you finish reading this first sequence, about 30 minutes from now, you'll know that losing weight is not complicated.

But that's not enough. You also have to want to lose it. And you have to decide what changes you will make.

We'll suggest plenty, but it's up to you to commit to a few.

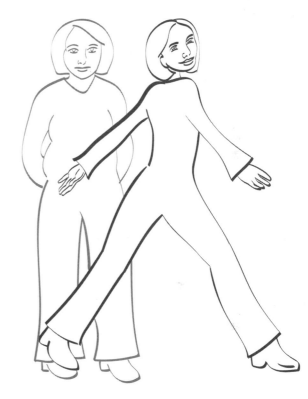

So how does your body gain and lose weight?

The science is straightforward. Food is the fuel your body uses to stay alive…

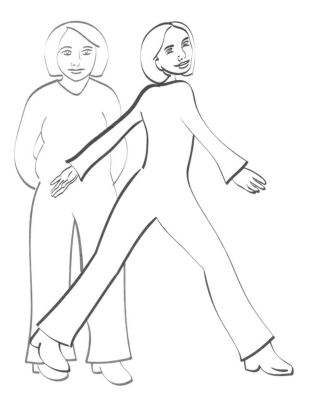

You put fuel in your car (1)…

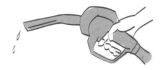

…and it is burned by the engine. The more driving you do, the more fuel you burn (2).

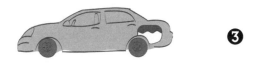

And whatever is left over has to go somewhere—in this case it simply stays in the tank (3).

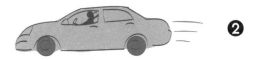

Similarly, your body converts food into fuel (1)…

…and burns what it needs. The more active you are, the more fuel your body burns (2).

Whatever is left over has to go somewhere—it is stored in your body (3).

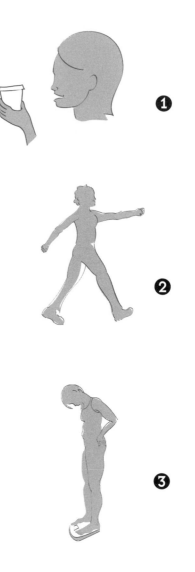

So if you eat more than your body burns, you will gain weight. If you eat less than you burn, you lose weight.

Simple as that.

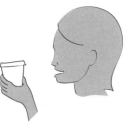

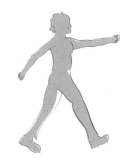

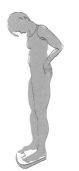

Let's take someone who eats
2,500 calories a day, on average.

(For comparison, a Big Mac has
600 calories.)

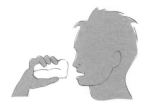

2,500 calories a day

Say they burn 2,000 calories a day—an average amount for someone who doesn't get a lot of exercise.

But 2,000 calories is 500 less than they are eating each day.

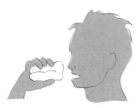

2,500 calories a day

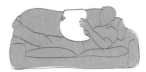

2,000 calories a day

500 calories a day is a key number for us. It equals one pound a week.

So someone who eats 500 calories a day more than they burn will gain one pound a week.

Every week.

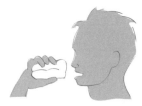

2,500 calories a day

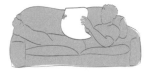

2,000 calories a day

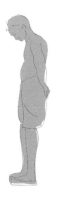

500 calories a day excess = 1 pound a week gain

Your turn.

If someone eats 3,000 calories a day and burns 2,000, how many pounds will their weight change by each week?

Don't flip the page until you are ready with an answer.

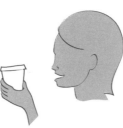

3,000 calories a day

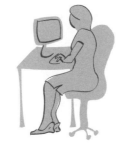

2,000 calories a day

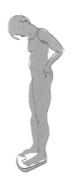

1,000 calories a day excess

They will gain two pounds
a week.

(This is a very important point.
If you didn't get it, take the time
to review the last few pages.)

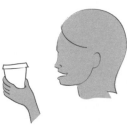

3,000 calories a day

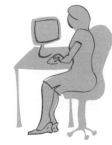

2,000 calories a day

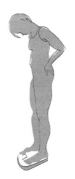

1000 calories a day excess
= 2 pounds a week gain

Now picture someone consuming 2,000 calories a day and burning the same amount. What will happen to their weight?

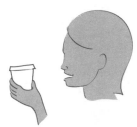

2,000 calories a day

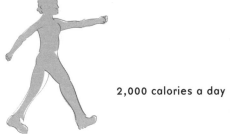

2,000 calories a day

It won't change.

Actually, short term it could fluctuate by as much as two pounds due to water retention. But medium and long term it will stay the same.

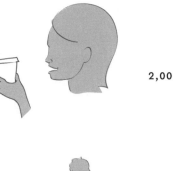

2,000 calories a day

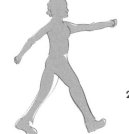

2,000 calories a day

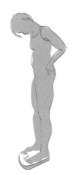

0 calories a day excess
= 0 pounds a week

Now let's take an athlete. They might burn much more energy, perhaps 3,500 calories a day.

If they eat more too—say 4,000 calories a day—what will happen to their weight?

(Here, and on the following pages, work out the actual number of pounds up or down per week.)

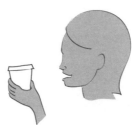

4,000 calories a day

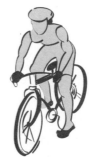

3,500 calories a day

They will add one pound a week, which is bad news (you don't see many obese athletes).

Athletes have to be very careful to take in the same amount of fuel as they burn, in this case 3,500 calories a day.

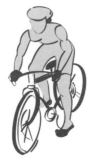

4,000 calories a day

3,500 calories a day

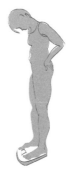

500 calories a day excess = 1 pound a week gain

3,500 calories, by the way, is
a lot of food. But if you burn a
lot, you can eat a lot.

So it doesn't matter how much
you eat. What matters is the
difference between how much
you eat and how much you burn.

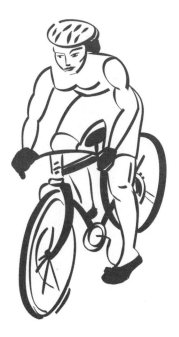

Here's a common story you may recognize.

Someone eats the same amount each day that they burn, say 2,000 calories. As we know, their weight stays the same.

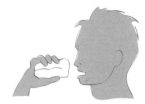

2,000 calories a day

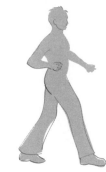

2,000 calories a day

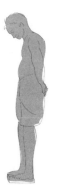

0 calories a day excess
= 0 pounds a week

But from the age of 30, the amount they burn starts to fall. Not much, perhaps to 1,750 calories a day.

This happens to everyone. Bodies actually burn less energy as they get older (like a more economical car, it burns less fuel for the same trip).

But what do you think happens to their weight (how many pounds up or down per week)?

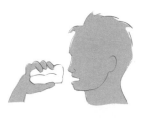

2,000 calories a day

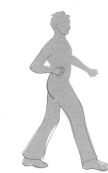

1,750 calories a day

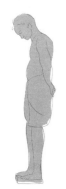

They start to gain weight slowly: half-a-pound every week.

After a year, they will have gained 26 pounds.

This is one reason why the proportion of overweight adults is four times higher than overweight teenagers.

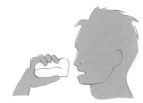

2,000 calories a day

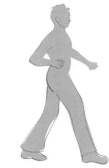

1,750 calories a day

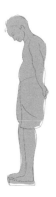

250 calories a day excess
= 1/2 pound a week gain

But now we can make this same equation work *for* us.

Say this same person wants to reduce their weight. They decide to replace a Big Mac and large Coke, which (let's say) they eat every day for lunch, with a Chicken McGrill and a diet Coke, which together contain 500 fewer calories.

So now they consume 1,500 calories a day and burn 1,750. What happens to their weight?

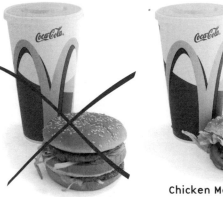

Big Mac = 600
Large Coke = 300

Chicken McGrill = 400
Diet Coke = 0

They lose half-a-pound each week, since they are eating 250 fewer calories a day than they are burning.

Notice that they lose weight even though they are still eating burgers—not the ideal lunch (we'll see exactly why later).

The *number of calories* matters more than where they come from.

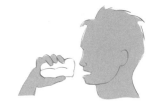

1,500 calories a day

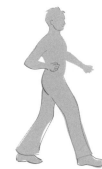

1,750 calories a day

250 calories a day saving
= 1/2 pound a week loss

Of course, if they reverse their decision, and start eating a Big Mac and large Coke again every day, they start putting weight back on.

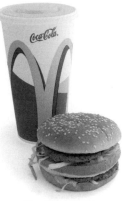

Big Mac = 600
Large Coke = 300

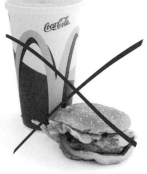

Chicken McGrill = 400
Diet Coke = 0

Which is exactly what happens to most people who diet; at some point, they go back to their old habits.

If you make a temporary change to your diet, you will get a temporary change in your body.

Your long-term habits dictate your weight. Small, long-term changes are what we are looking for.

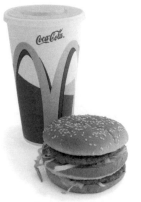

Big Mac = 600
Large Coke = 300

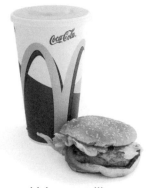

Chicken McGrill = 400
Diet Coke = 0

The changes that cause you to gain weight—such as getting older, quitting smoking, pregnancy—have long-term effects.

So the changes you need to make in response must be long-term too.

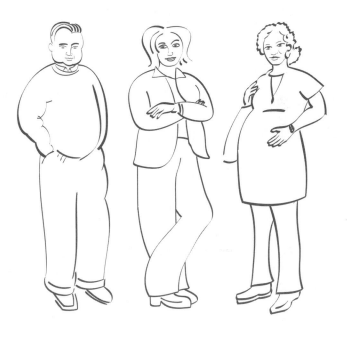

But how easy is it to cut 500 calories a day? To find out, let's look at some more examples.

Super Size french fries are a massive 600 calories, the same as a Big Mac. Medium french fries are 450.

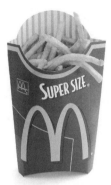

Super Size french fries = 600

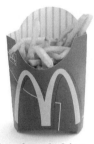

Medium french fries = 450

How many calories do you think there are in a small french fries?

Take a guess before flipping the page—it will help you remember.

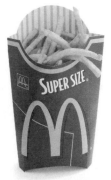

Super Size french fries = 600

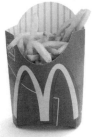

Medium french fries = 450

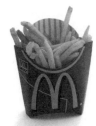

Small french fries = ?

Only 200.

So, every time you substitute small for medium french fries, you save 250 calories—half the daily target.

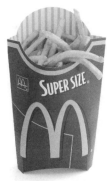

Super Size french fries = 600

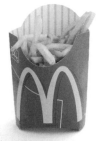

Medium french fries = 450

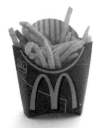

Small french fries = 200

A large Coca-Cola is 300 calories. How many calories would you estimate for a standard, 12-ounce can of Coca-Cola?

(Hint: the can contains about half as much coke.)

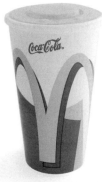

Large Coca-Cola = 300

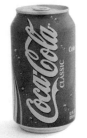

12-oz Coca-Cola = ?

150.

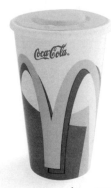

Large Coca-Cola = 300

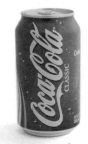

12-oz Coca-Cola = 150

And how many in a can of Pepsi?

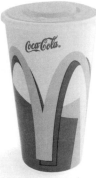

Large Coca-Cola = 300

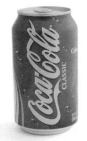

12-oz Coca-Cola = 150

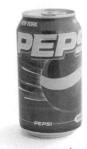

12-oz Pepsi = ?

150 again.

Same for Sprite, Seven-Up, Mountain Dew, and Ginger Ale. In fact, just about any 12-ounce can of soda.

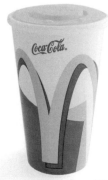

Large Coca-Cola = 300

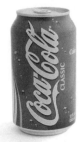

12-oz Coca-Cola = 150

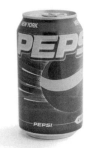

12-oz Pepsi = 150

How many calories would you
estimate for a 12-ounce bottle
of Budweiser?

Take a guess.

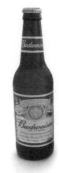

Also 150. Same for a bottle of Coors, Miller, Heineken, etc.

Same too for a typical glass of wine (white or red), a shot of whisky, or a gin and tonic —the calories are in the alcohol.

Smaller glasses or weaker drinks have fewer calories (light beers, for instance, are around 120). Large glasses have more. Doubles have, well, double.

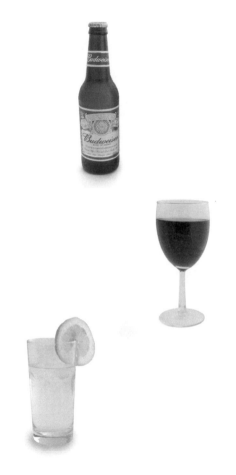

What about a plain old cup of coffee or tea?

Make your estimate before flipping the page. Assume no milk or sugar.

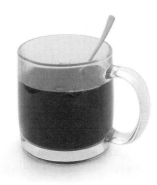

0.

(Well, 3 calories actually, but that's close enough to zero for our purposes.)

Half and half adds 75 calories, whole milk adds 50, skim milk adds 25.

And 15 calories for each teaspoon of sugar.

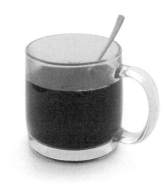

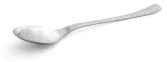

So if you drink 5 cups of coffee a day, each with 2 teaspoons of sugar, that's 10 teaspoons of sugar per day.

Say you cut out the sugar, or substitute a zero-calorie sweetener such as Extra or NutraSweet. How many calories are you saving each day by cutting out 10 teaspoons of sugar?

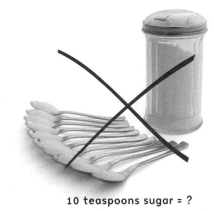

10 teaspoons sugar = ?

150.

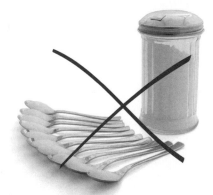

10 teaspoons sugar = 10 x 15 = 150

If you used to drink three cans of Coca-Cola a day and you substitute Diet Coke for all three, how many calories are you saving?

Don't flip the page without trying to answer (unless you really have to).

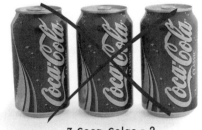

3 Coca-Colas = ?

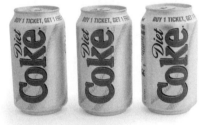

3 Diet Cokes = ?

3 x 150 = 450. Almost an entire 500 calorie daily target.

(If you've been avoiding diet sodas because of cancer concerns around saccharin, don't worry: most diet drinks, and both NutraSweet and Equal, use aspartame, which dozens of studies have found to be safe.)

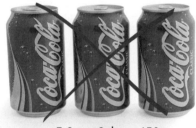

3 Coca-Colas = 450

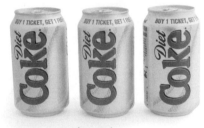

3 Diet Cokes = 0

Of course, you may say that diet soda, or coffee without sugar, tastes worse.

But tastes can be acquired. Few people like beer the first time they taste it and many people love the taste of raw fish.

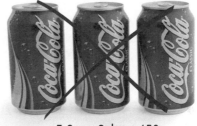

3 Coca-Colas = 450

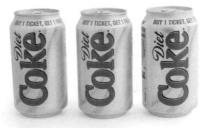

3 Diet Cokes = 0

Making a permanent substitution often means modifying your tastes (something most short-term diets fail to point out).

In fact, after switching to a new taste for four weeks or more, you will most likely find it odd going back to the old one.

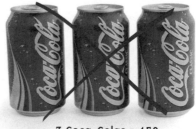

3 Coca-Colas = 450

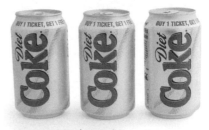

3 Diet Cokes = 0

Another substitution: instead of ordering Super Size fries you order small. How many calories do you save?

Answer without flipping back if you can.

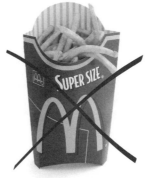
Super Size fries = ?

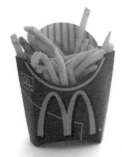
Small fries = ?

600 - 200 = 400.

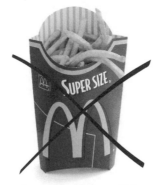
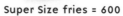

Super Size fries = 600

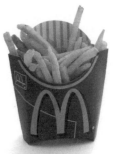

Small fries = 200

Let's look at some typical snacks.

A single Snickers has around 250 calories. How many calories do you think are in a pack of Reese's Peanut Butter Cups?

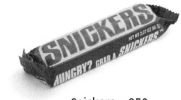

Snickers = 250

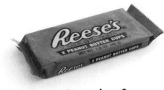

Reese's = ?

250.

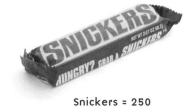

Snickers = 250

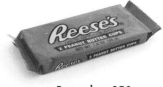

Reese's = 250

How many in a pack of M&Ms?

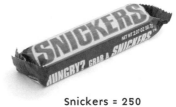

Snickers = 250

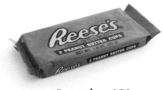

Reese's = 250

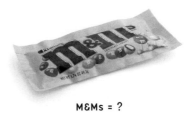

M&Ms = ?

250.

Same for Twix, Milky Way,
3 Musketeers, Kit Kat,
Butterfinger and just about
any standard size candy bar.

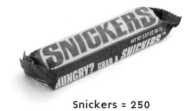

Snickers = 250

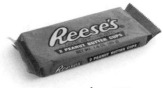

Reese's = 250

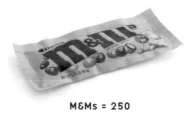

M&Ms = 250

For the same 250 calories, you can get a whole meal from—get ready for this—McDonald's.

A Grilled Chicken Caesar Salad *with low-fat dressing* has the same number of calories as a single candy bar.

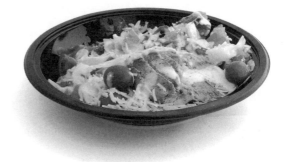

(Other dressings contain a lot more calories, maybe even more than the salad.)

A bagel is also 250…

…but only if you don't put anything on it: cream cheese adds another 250, making 500.

Often, what you put on food contains as many calories as what you put it on—dressing on salad, butter and jam on toast, etc.

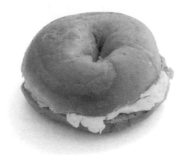

The typical muffin, such as you would find at Dunkin Donuts or Starbucks, is a cool 500 calories.

Some muffins are as much as 800.

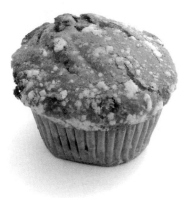

While we're at Starbucks, let's look at coffee drinks with a high milk content such as a latte, cappuccino, or frappuccino.

The calories in coffee are in the milk (and sugar, if you add it) as we already noted.

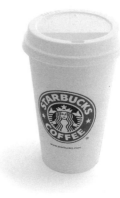

So there's a great substitution here: choose non-fat milk instead of whole milk in a grande and save around 100 calories.

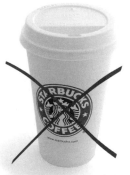

Whole milk grande latte

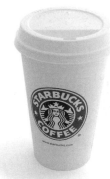

Non-fat grande latte
save 100 calories

Even better, switch from grande to tall as well and save another 50—tall is, after all, not small.

In fact, serving sizes have grown larger and larger, at about the same rate as the average waist. A Super Size soda contains more than two whole cans (and more than 400 calories). Does anyone really need that much in one drink?

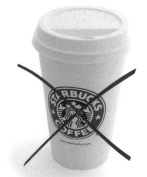

Whole milk grande latte

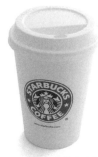

Non-fat tall latte save 150 calories

Does your stomach know when to stop eating? Yes, but there's a problem.

Your body sends satiety ("suh-TIE-a-tee") signals to your brain—saying, "Hey, I'm full"—but these can arrive 15 minutes or more after you really were full.

By then you may have overeaten.

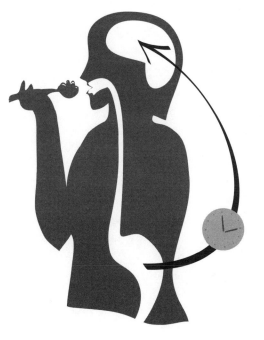

So a good rule is to stop eating *before* you're completely full, even if that means leaving some food (you'll know to order less next time).

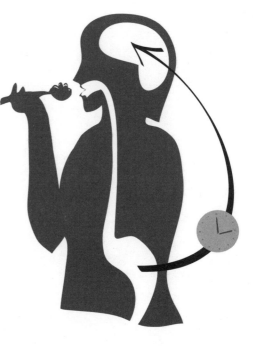

Likewise, don't eat if you're not hungry. You'll enjoy it far more when you are.

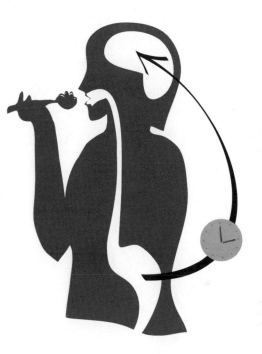

Hunger and satiety mechanisms were evolved by your distant ancestors when food was tough to come by. (When stone age man scraped together his dinner, no-one asked if he wanted to Super Size it.)

Your ancestors also evolved a taste for sweet things, perhaps to tell them which foods were quick sources of energy. Which helps explain why tempting food left around tends to get eaten.

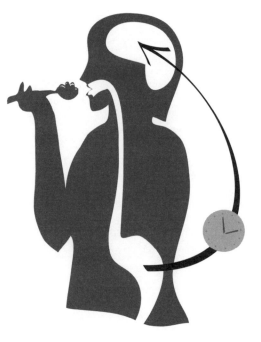

These mechanisms were never intended to fine-tune your nutritional intake in 21st century America, where food is not tough to come by.

The result is that your body builds an 'emergency' store of energy (fat, in other words) for an emergency that never arrives.

We need to learn some new tactics…

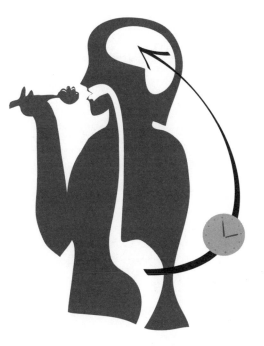

Three helpful tactics are:

1. Stop eating *before* you are full.

2. Don't eat if you're not hungry.

3. Avoid leaving tempting food around.

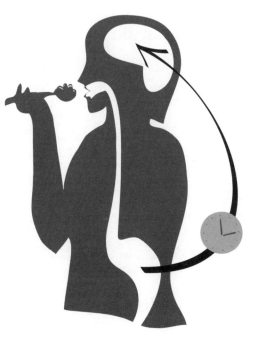

So far we've looked at high-calorie snacks—not because anyone would recommend them, of course, but so you know what you're eating.

Nature provides an ideal alternative snack (though she neglected to provide an advertising budget): fruit.

A single piece of any of these fruits is just 50 calories —except one. Any idea which?

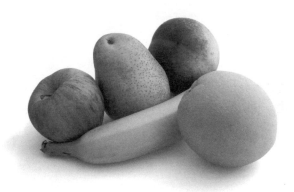

The banana.

It has more calories than any other fruit, but still not excessive at 100.

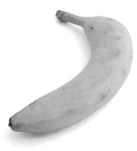

Which has more calories, do you think, a banana or a slice of toast with margarine?

Stop and think about it before flipping the page.

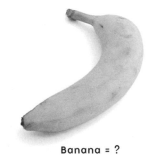

Banana = ?

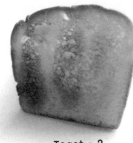

Toast = ?

In fact, both are about the same,
100 calories.

You may find that an
unexpectedly high energy
content for a single slice of
bread. And it's even higher if
you lace it with jam.

('Energy' and 'calories' are the
same thing, by the way.)

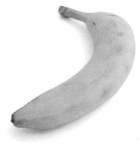

Banana = 100

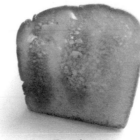

Toast = 100

Vegetables are famously low
in calories.

How many in a stick of celery?
Take a guess.

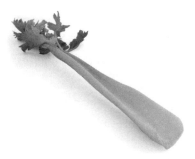

5.

In fact, you use as much energy
eating a stick of celery as there is
in it, so you can eat as many
sticks as you want.

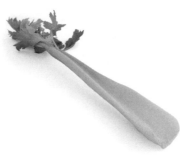

A little recap.

How many calories in a Grilled
Chicken Caesar Salad?

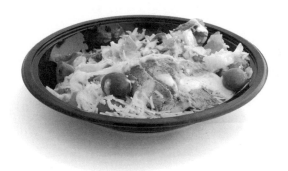

250.

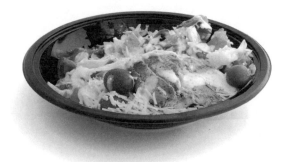

How many in a bagel with
cream cheese?

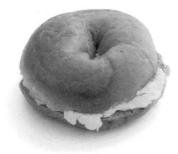

500.

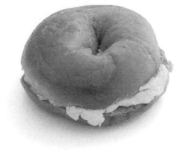

How many calories do you save
by substituting a non-fat tall
latte for a whole milk grande?

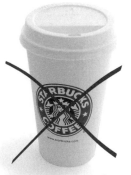

Whole milk grande latte

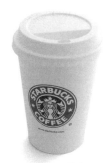

**Non-fat tall latte
save ? calories**

150.

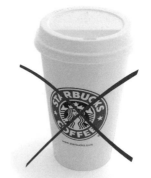

Whole milk grande latte

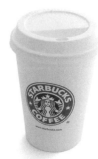

Non-fat tall latte
save 150 calories

Do you remember the number
of calories in a Big Mac?

(Hint: it's the same as the
number of calories in Super Size
french fries.)

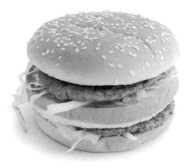

600.

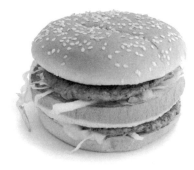

And how many calories a day do you need to save in order to lose one pound a week?

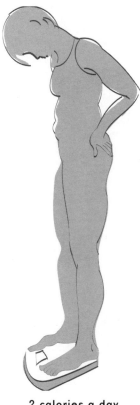

? calories a day
= 1 pound a week

500.

Now may be a good time to figure out how long it would take you to reach your target weight (from page 9) assuming you lose a pound a week.

Some readers find it helps to work out the actual date they could reach their target.

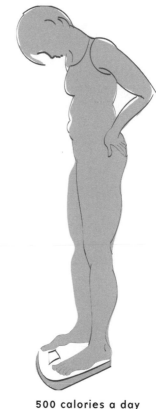

500 calories a day = 1 pound a week

The calories in many snacks can be difficult to gauge.

Take this 5½-ounce bag of potato chips. Here is the Nutrition Facts label on the bag.

How many calories would you consume if you ate it?

Nutrition Facts

Serving Size 1 oz (28g/About 20 chips)
Servings Per Container About 6

Amount Per Serving

Calories 150	Calories from Fat 90

	% Daily Value*
Total Fat 10g	**15%**
Saturated Fat 3g	**15%**
Cholesterol 0mg	**0%**
Sodium 180mg	**8%**
Total Carbohydrate 15g	**5%**
Dietary Fiber 1g	**4%**
Sugars 0g	
Protein 2g	

Vitamin A 0%	•	Vitamin C 10%
Calcuim 0%	•	Iron 0%

* Percent Daily Values are based on a 2,000 calorie diet. Your daily values may be higher or lower depending on your calorie needs:

	Calories:	2,000	2,500
Total Fat	Less than	65g	80g
Sat Fat	Less than	20g	25g
Cholesterol	Less than	300mg	300mg
Sodium	Less than	2,400mg	2,400mg
Total Carbohydrate		300g	375g
Dietary Fiber		25g	30g

Calories per gram: Fat 9 • Carbohydrate 4 • Protein 4

150 right? Wrong.

150 is a single serving. But this bag has been deemed to contain six servings. So the whole bag is 150 x 6 = 900 calories.

When was the last time you ate only one sixth of a bag of Lays?

Nutrition Facts

Serving Size 1 oz (28g/About 20 chips)
Servings Per Container About 6

Amount Per Serving

Calories 150	Calories from Fat 90

	% Daily Value*
Total Fat 10g	**15**%
Saturated Fat 3g	**15**%
Cholesterol 0mg	**0**%
Sodium 180mg	**8**%
Total Carbohydrate 15g	**5**%
Dietary Fiber 1g	**4**%
Sugars 0g	
Protein 2g	

Vitamin A 0%	•	Vitamin C 10%
Calcuim 0%	•	Iron 0%

* Percent Daily Values are based on a 2,000 calorie diet.
Your daily values may be higher or lower depending
on your calorie needs:

		Calories:	2,000	2,500
Total Fat	Less than		65g	80g
Sat Fat	Less than		20g	25g
Cholesterol	Less than		300mg	300mg
Sodium	Less than		2,400mg	2,400mg
Total Carbohydrate			300g	375g
Dietary Fiber			25g	30g

Calories per gram: Fat 9 • Carbohydrate 4 • Protein 4

It seems odd, when most servings are getting larger, that serving sizes on labels are almost always too small.

Cynics might say this is so manufacturers can claim that each serving has only a small number of calories.

Nutrition Facts

Serving Size 1 oz (28g/About 20 chips)
Servings Per Container About 6

Amount Per Serving

Calories 150   Calories from Fat 90

	% Daily Value*
Total Fat 10g	**15%**
Saturated Fat 3g	**15%**
Cholesterol 0mg	**0%**
Sodium 180mg	**8%**
Total Carbohydrate 15g	**5%**
Dietary Fiber 1g	**4%**
Sugars 0g	
Protein 2g	

Vitamin A 0%	•	Vitamin C 10%
Calcuim 0%	•	Iron 0%

*Percent Daily Values are based on a 2,000 calorie diet. Your daily values may be higher or lower depending on your calorie needs:

	Calories:	2,000	2,500
Total Fat	Less than	65g	80g
Sat Fat	Less than	20g	25g
Cholesterol	Less than	300mg	300mg
Sodium	Less than	2,400mg	2,400mg
Total Carbohydrate		300g	375g
Dietary Fiber		25g	30g

Calories per gram: Fat 9 • Carbohydrate 4 • Protein 4

There is a lot of information on Nutrition Facts labels—maybe too much.

In practice, only five numbers are usually worth a look: the serving size, number of calories, and three others we'll come to later.

Nutrition Facts

Serving Size 1 oz (28g/About 20 chips)
Servings Per Container About 6

Amount Per Serving		
Calories 150	Calories from Fat 90	

		% Daily Value*
Total Fat 10g		**15%**
Saturated Fat 3g		**15%**
Cholesterol 0mg		**0%**
Sodium 180mg		**8%**
Total Carbohydrate 15g		**5%**
Dietary Fiber 1g		**4%**
Sugars 0g		
Protein 2g		

Vitamin A 0%	•	Vitamin C 10%	
Calcuim 0%	•	Iron 0%	

*Percent Daily Values are based on a 2,000 calorie diet. Your daily values may be higher or lower depending on your calorie needs:

	Calories:	2,000	2,500
Total Fat	Less than	65g	80g
Sat Fat	Less than	20g	25g
Cholesterol	Less than	300mg	300mg
Sodium	Less than	2,400mg	2,400mg
Total Carbohydrate		300g	375g
Dietary Fiber		25g	30g

Calories per gram: Fat 9 • Carbohydrate 4 • Protein 4

Let's try another. Here is a pint of ice cream.

How many calories in one serving (½ cup)?

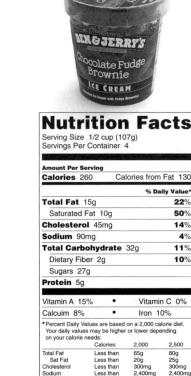

Nutrition Facts

Serving Size 1/2 cup (107g)
Servings Per Container 4

Amount Per Serving

Calories 260	Calories from Fat 130

	% Daily Value*
Total Fat 15g	**22**%
Saturated Fat 10g	**50**%
Cholesterol 45mg	**14**%
Sodium 90mg	**4**%
Total Carbohydrate 32g	**11**%
Dietary Fiber 2g	**10**%
Sugars 27g	
Protein 5g	

Vitamin A 15%	•	Vitamin C 0%
Calcuim 8%	•	Iron 10%

*Percent Daily Values are based on a 2,000 calorie diet.
Your daily values may be higher or lower depending
on your calorie needs:

	Calories:	2,000	2,500
Total Fat	Less than	65g	80g
Sat Fat	Less than	20g	25g
Cholesterol	Less than	300mg	300mg
Sodium	Less than	2,400mg	2,400mg
Total Carbohydrate		300g	375g
Dietary Fiber		25g	30g

Calories per gram: Fat 9 • Carbohydrate 4 • Protein 4

260.

Nutrition Facts

Serving Size 1/2 cup (107g)
Servings Per Container 4

Amount Per Serving

Calories 260   Calories from Fat 130

	% Daily Value*
Total Fat 15g	**22%**
Saturated Fat 10g	**50%**
Cholesterol 45mg	**14%**
Sodium 90mg	**4%**
Total Carbohydrate 32g	**11%**
Dietary Fiber 2g	**10%**
Sugars 27g	
Protein 5g	

Vitamin A 15%	•	Vitamin C 0%
Calcium 8%	•	Iron 10%

*Percent Daily Values are based on a 2,000 calorie diet.
Your daily values may be higher or lower depending
on your calorie needs:

	Calories:	2,000	2,500
Total Fat	Less than	65g	80g
Sat Fat	Less than	20g	25g
Cholesterol	Less than	300mg	300mg
Sodium	Less than	2,400mg	2,400mg
Total Carbohydrate		300g	375g
Dietary Fiber		25g	30g

Calories per gram: Fat 9 • Carbohydrate 4 • Protein 4

Here's a different tub.

How many calories would you consume in one serving of this ice cream?

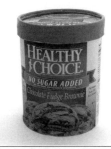

Nutrition Facts

Serving Size 1/2 cup (71g)
Servings Per Container 14

Amount Per Serving

Calories 120	Calories from Fat 20

	% Daily Value*
Total Fat 2g	**3**%
Saturated Fat 1g	**5**%
Polyunsaturated Fat 0g	
Monounsaturated Fat 0.5g	
Cholesterol 5mg	**2**%
Sodium 60mg	**3**%
Total Carbohydrate 21g	**7**%
Dietary Fiber 1g	**4**%
Sugars 4g	
Sugar Alcohols 7g	
Protein 3g	

Vitamin A 4%	•	Vitamin C 0%
Calcuim 10%	•	Iron 0%

*Percent Daily Values are based on a 2,000 calorie diet.
Your daily values may be higher or lower depending
on your calorie needs:

		Calories:	2,000	2,500
Total Fat	Less than		65g	80g
Sat Fat	Less than		20g	25g
Cholesterol	Less than		300mg	300mg
Sodium	Less than		2,400mg	2,400mg
Total Carbohydrate			300g	375g
Dietary Fiber			25g	30g

Calories per gram: Fat 9 • Carbohydrate 4 • Protein 4

120.

Less than half the Ben & Jerry's.

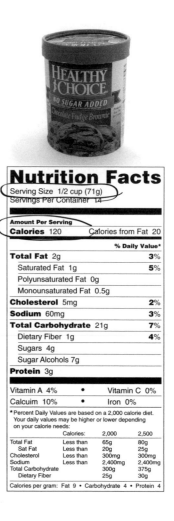

When you start looking at the labels, you'll find some things that may surprise you.

For instance, how many calories would you consume by eating just 39 peanuts from this bag?

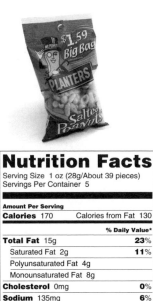

Nutrition Facts

Serving Size 1 oz (28g/About 39 pieces)
Servings Per Container 5

Amount Per Serving

Calories 170   Calories from Fat 130

	% Daily Value*
Total Fat 15g	**23**%
Saturated Fat 2g	**11**%
Polyunsaturated Fat 4g	
Monounsaturated Fat 8g	
Cholesterol 0mg	**0**%
Sodium 135mg	**6**%
Potassium 190mg	**5**%
Total Carbohydrate 5g	**2**%
Dietary Fiber 2g	**9**%
Sugars less than 1g	
Protein 7g	**7**%

Vitamin A 0%	•	Vitamin C 0%
Calcuim 0%	•	Iron 2%

*Percent Daily Values are based on a 2,000 calorie diet.
Your daily values may be higher or lower depending
on your calorie needs:

		Calories:	2,000	2,500
Total Fat	Less than		65g	80g
Sat Fat	Less than		20g	25g
Cholesterol	Less than		300mg	300mg
Sodium	Less than		2,400mg	2,400mg
Total Carbohydrate			300g	375g
Dietary Fiber			25g	30g

Calories per gram: Fat 9 • Carbohydrate 4 • Protein 4

170. If you ate the whole 5-ounce bag, that would be 850 calories!

Peanuts are a good example of a high energy food: they are little bullets of calories.

So the peanuts you nibble before a meal could contain nearly as many calories as the meal itself.

Nutrition Facts

Serving Size 1 oz (28g/About 39 pieces)
Servings Per Container 5

Amount Per Serving

Calories 170   Calories from Fat 130

	% Daily Value*
Total Fat 15g	**23%**
Saturated Fat 2g	**11%**
Polyunsaturated Fat 4g	
Monounsaturated Fat 8g	
Cholesterol 0mg	**0%**
Sodium 135mg	**6%**
Potassium 190mg	**5%**
Total Carbohydrate 5g	**2%**
Dietary Fiber 2g	**9%**
Sugars less than 1g	
Protein 7g	**7%**

Vitamin A 0%	•	Vitamin C 0%	
Calcuim 0%	•	Iron 2%	

* Percent Daily Values are based on a 2,000 calorie diet.
Your daily values may be higher or lower depending on your calorie needs:

		Calories:	2,000	2,500
Total Fat	Less than		65g	80g
Sat Fat	Less than		20g	25g
Cholesterol	Less than		300mg	300mg
Sodium	Less than		2,400mg	2,400mg
Total Carbohydrate			300g	375g
Dietary Fiber			25g	30g

Calories per gram: Fat 9 • Carbohydrate 4 • Protein 4

Now some recap questions
before we round out Sequence
One. See if you can answer them
without turning back.

How much energy is there in an
apple? (Remember, 'energy'
means the same as 'calories'.)

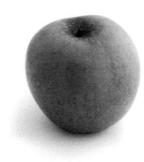

50.

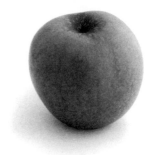

How much in this can of soda?

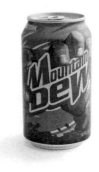

150.

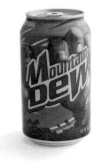

And how much in this candy bar?

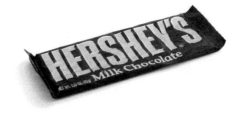

250.

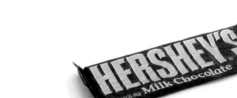

You can use your knowledge of one food to estimate the calories in dozens of others.

For instance, each Hershey's Kiss in this bag is roughly one tenth of a candy bar.

So how much energy in a single Kiss?

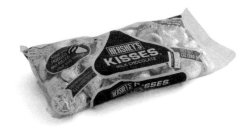

$250 \div 10 = 25.$

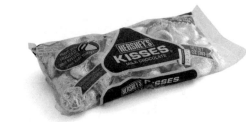

Which of these two types of 'health' bars has fewer calories per bar?

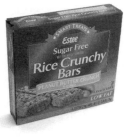

Nutrition Facts

Serving Size 1 Bar (19g)
Servings Per Container 4

Amount Per Serving

Calories 70	Calories from Fat 10

	% Daily Value*
Total Fat 1g	**2**%
Sodium 35mg	**1**%
Total Carbohydrate 15g	**5**%
Sugar Alcohol 8g	
Protein 1g	

Not a significant source of saturated fat, cholesterol, dietary fiber, sugars, vitamin A, vitamin C, calcium, and iron.

*Percent Daily Values are based on a 2,000 calorie diet. Your daily values may be higher or lower depending on your calorie needs:

		Calories:	2,000	2,500
Total Fat	Less than		65g	80g
Sat Fat	Less than		20g	25g
Cholesterol	Less than		300mg	300mg
Sodium	Less than		2,400mg	2,400mg
Total Carbohydrate			300g	375g
Dietary Fiber			25g	30g

Calories per gram: Fat 9 • Carbohydrate 4 • Protein 4

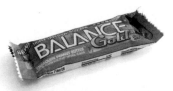

Nutrition Facts

Serving Size 1 bar (50g)
Calories 210
Calories from Fat 60
*Percent Daily Values (DV) are based on a 2,000 calorie diet.

Amount/Serving	%DV*	Amount/Serving	%DV*
Total Fat 7g	**11**%	**Total Carbohydrate** 22g	**7**%
Saturated Fat 4g	**20**%	Dietary Fiber <1g	**3**%
Cholesterol 0mg	**0**%	Sugars 11g	
Sodium 125mg	**5**%	**Protein** 15g	
Potassium 125mg	**4**%		

Vitamin A 50% (99% as beta-carotene)	• Vitamin C 100%	• Calcium 10%	• Iron 25%	• Vitamin E 100%	
Vitamin K 25%	• Thiamin 25%	• Riboflavin 25%	• Niacin 25%	• Vitamin B6 25%	• Folic Acid 25%
Vitamin B12 25%	• Biotin 25%	• Pantothenic Acid 25%	• Phosphorus 15%	• Iodine 25%	• Magnesium 10%
Zinc 25%	• Selenium 25%	• Copper 25%	• Manganese 25%	• Chromium 25%	• Molybdenum 25%

The one at the top: 70 calories.

The other has a similar number of calories as a Snickers, which is not normally considered a health bar!

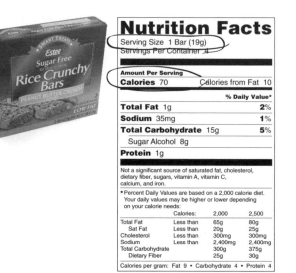

Nutrition Facts

Serving Size 1 Bar (19g)
Servings Per Container 4

Amount Per Serving

Calories 70   Calories from Fat 10

	% Daily Value*
Total Fat 1g	**2%**
Sodium 35mg	**1%**
Total Carbohydrate 15g	**5%**
Sugar Alcohol 8g	
Protein 1g	

Not a significant source of saturated fat, cholesterol, dietary fiber, sugars, vitamin A, vitamin C, calcium, and iron.

*Percent Daily Values are based on a 2,000 calorie diet. Your daily values may be higher or lower depending on your calorie needs:

		Calories:	2,000	2,500
Total Fat	Less than		65g	80g
Sat Fat	Less than		20g	25g
Cholesterol	Less than		300mg	300mg
Sodium	Less than		2,400mg	2,400mg
Total Carbohydrate			300g	375g
Dietary Fiber			25g	30g

Calories per gram: Fat 9 • Carbohydrate 4 • Protein 4

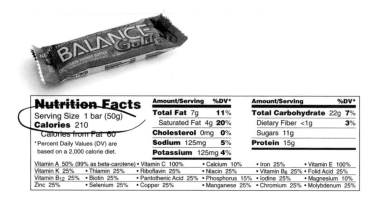

Nutrition Facts

Serving Size 1 bar (50g)
Calories 210
Calories from Fat 60
*Percent Daily Values (DV) are based on a 2,000 calorie diet.

Amount/Serving	%DV*	Amount/Serving	%DV*
Total Fat 7g	**11%**	**Total Carbohydrate** 22g	**7%**
Saturated Fat 4g	**20%**	Dietary Fiber <1g	**3%**
Cholesterol 0mg	**0%**	Sugars 11g	
Sodium 125mg	**5%**	**Protein** 15g	
Potassium 125mg	**4%**		

Vitamin A 50% (99% as beta-carotene)	• Vitamin C 100%	• Calcium 10%	• Iron 25%	• Vitamin E 100%	
Vitamin K 25%	• Thiamin 25%	• Riboflavin 25%	• Niacin 25%	• Vitamin B6 25%	• Folid Acid 25%
Vitamin B12 25%	• Biotin 25%	• Pantothenic Acid 25%	• Phosphorus 15%	• Iodine 25%	• Magnesium 10%
Zinc 25%	• Selenium 25%	• Copper 25%	• Manganese 25%	• Chromium 25%	• Molybdenum 25%

If you were going to make only one of these two substitutions, which saves more calories:

- Drink water instead of a can of soda, or

- Eat an apple instead of a candy bar?

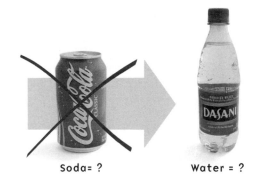

Soda= ?   Water = ?

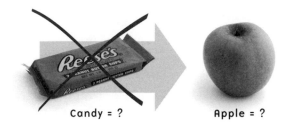

Candy = ?   Apple = ?

Eating an apple instead of a candy bar is the better substitution, replacing 250 calories with 50, and saving 200.

(A can of soda is 150 and water is zero, so this substitution is also a good one at 150 calories.)

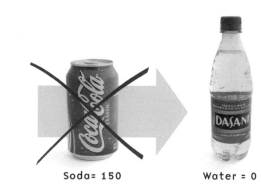

Soda= 150   Water = 0

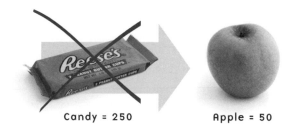

Candy = 250   Apple = 50

And which of these two substitutions saves more calories:

- Drink water instead of a can of soda, or

- Eat a slice of toast instead of a cream cheese bagel?

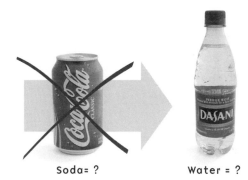

Soda= ?   Water = ?

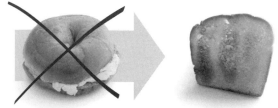

Cream cheese bagel = ?   Toast = ?

Eating a slice of toast instead of a cream cheese bagel saves more —replacing 500 calories with 100, saving 400.

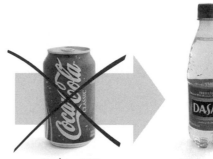

Soda= 150   Water = 0

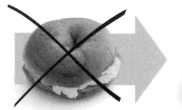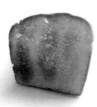

Cream cheese bagel = 500   Toast = 100

Which of these two bags contains fewer calories per serving, the classic chips or the reduced fat chips?

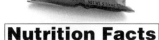

Nutrition Facts

Serving Size 1 oz (28g/About 20 chips)
Servings Per Container About 6

Amount Per Serving

Calories 150	Calories from Fat 90

	% Daily Value*
Total Fat 10g	**15%**
Saturated Fat 3g	**15%**
Cholesterol 0mg	**0%**
Sodium 180mg	**8%**
Total Carbohydrate 15g	**5%**
Dietary Fiber 1g	**4%**
Sugars 0g	
Protein 2g	

Vitamin A 0%	•	Vitamin C 10%
Calcuim 0%	•	Iron 0%

*Percent Daily Values are based on a 2,000 calorie diet. Your daily values may be higher or lower depending on your calorie needs:

	Calories:	2,000	2,500
Total Fat	Less than	65g	80g
Sat Fat	Less than	20g	25g
Cholesterol	Less than	300mg	300mg
Sodium	Less than	2,400mg	2,400mg
Total Carbohydrate		300g	375g
Dietary Fiber		25g	30g

Calories per gram: Fat 9 • Carbohydrate 4 • Protein 4

Nutrition Facts

Serving Size 1 oz (28g/About 14 chips)
Servings Per Container 8

Amount Per Serving

Calories 140	Calories from Fat 60

	% Daily Value*
Total Fat 7g	**10%**
Saturated Fat 0.5g	**3%**
Cholesterol 0mg	**0%**
Sodium 160mg	**6%**
Total Carbohydrate 17g	**6%**
Dietary Fiber 1g	**5%**
Sugars 0g	
Protein 2g	

Vitamin A 0%	•	Vitamin C 10%
Calcuim 0%	•	Iron 2%
Vitamin E 10%	•	Thiamin 2%
Niacin 6%	•	Vitamin B6 4%
Phosphorus 4%	•	Zinc 2%

*Percent Daily Values are based on a 2,000 calorie diet. Your daily values may be higher or lower depending on your calorie needs:

	Calories:	2,000	2,500
Total Fat	Less than	65g	80g
Sat Fat	Less than	20g	25g
Cholesterol	Less than	300mg	300mg
Sodium	Less than	2,400mg	2,400mg
Total Carbohydrate		300g	375g
Dietary Fiber		25g	30g

Calories per gram: Fat 9 • Carbohydrate 4 • Protein 4

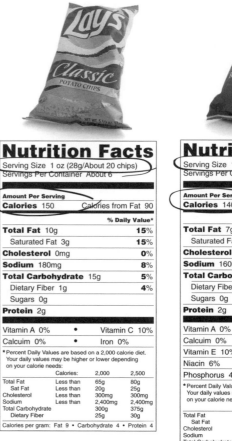

The reduced fat chips.

But, surprisingly, only just:
140 calories versus 150.

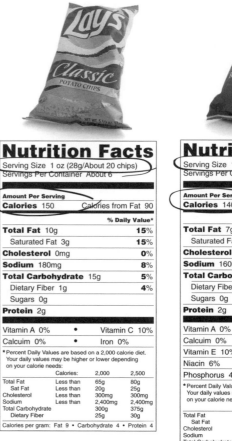

Nutrition Facts

Serving Size 1 oz (28g/About 20 chips)
Servings Per Container About 6

Amount Per Serving
Calories 150   Calories from Fat 90

	% Daily Value*
Total Fat 10g	**15%**
Saturated Fat 3g	**15%**
Cholesterol 0mg	**0%**
Sodium 180mg	**8%**
Total Carbohydrate 15g	**5%**
Dietary Fiber 1g	**4%**
Sugars 0g	
Protein 2g	

Vitamin A 0%	•	Vitamin C 10%
Calcuim 0%	•	Iron 0%

*Percent Daily Values are based on a 2,000 calorie diet. Your daily values may be higher or lower depending on your calorie needs:

	Calories:	2,000	2,500
Total Fat	Less than	65g	80g
Sat Fat	Less than	20g	25g
Cholesterol	Less than	300mg	300mg
Sodium	Less than	2,400mg	2,400mg
Total Carbohydrate		300g	375g
Dietary Fiber		25g	30g

Calories per gram: Fat 9 • Carbohydrate 4 • Protein 4

Nutrition Facts

Serving Size 1 oz (28g/About 14 chips)
Servings Per Container 8

Amount Per Serving
Calories 140   Calories from Fat 60

	% Daily Value*
Total Fat 7g	**10%**
Saturated Fat 0.5g	**3%**
Cholesterol 0mg	**0%**
Sodium 160mg	**6%**
Total Carbohydrate 17g	**6%**
Dietary Fiber 1g	**5%**
Sugars 0g	
Protein 2g	

Vitamin A 0%	•	Vitamin C 10%
Calcuim 0%	•	Iron 2%
Vitamin E 10%	•	Thiamin 2%
Niacin 6%	•	Vitamin B6 4%
Phosphorus 4%	•	Zinc 2%

*Percent Daily Values are based on a 2,000 calorie diet. Your daily values may be higher or lower depending on your calorie needs:

	Calories:	2,000	2,500
Total Fat	Less than	65g	80g
Sat Fat	Less than	20g	25g
Cholesterol	Less than	300mg	300mg
Sodium	Less than	2,400mg	2,400mg
Total Carbohydrate		300g	375g
Dietary Fiber		25g	30g

Calories per gram: Fat 9 • Carbohydrate 4 • Protein 4

Name any one of the three
tactics you can use to improve
your body's hunger and
satiety signals.

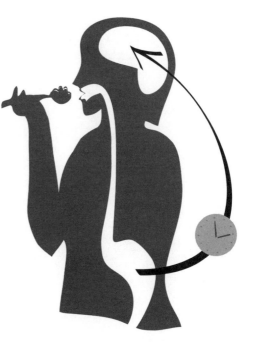

The three tactics are:

1. Stop eating *before* you are full.

2. Don't eat if you're not hungry.

3. Avoid leaving tempting food around.

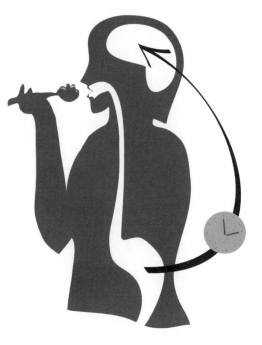

If you got these right, you're on your way to being a weight management practitioner. Congratulations!

If not, now may be a good time to go back and review anything you missed.

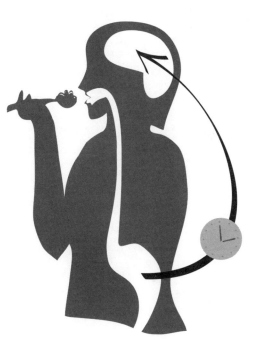

Reducing what you consume is only one side of weight management, of course. The other is burning more through exercise, which we'll cover in Sequence Two.

But you already know enough to take control of your weight right away.

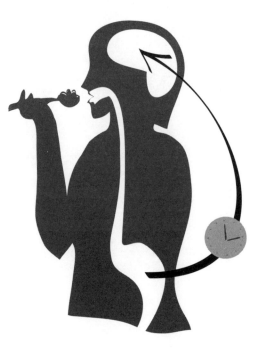

For instance, if you wanted to lose one pound a week, you could start by cutting your intake by 500 calories a day using the substitutions we have covered, or any of your own.

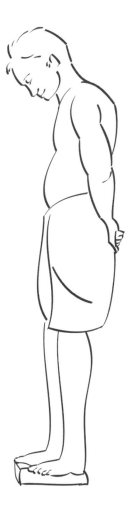

Remember, we are looking for substitutions that you are willing to make long term, not short-term sacrifices.

For this reason, some people find it easier to start by cutting 250 calories a day, though their progress will be a bit slower.

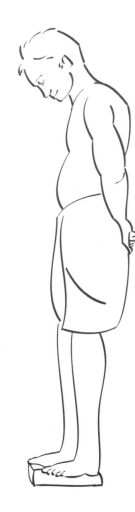

A substitution could mean replacing something you eat regularly with a *lower-energy alternative*.

Or eating the same things but *not as often*.

Or eating the same things just as often but *smaller amounts* of them.

Whole   Skim

Two per day   One per day

Grande   Tall

In trying to alter your weight, it's important that you measure your progress on a scale, or else you won't know whether you are succeeding.

Weigh yourself at least once a week at the same time of day —first thing in the morning is best. Wear as little as possible.

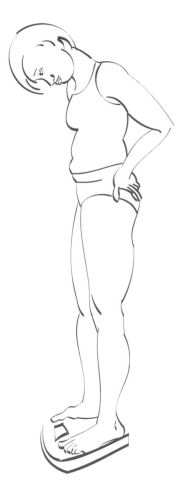

If 500 calories a day translates into one pound a week, will you see a result one week from now?

Perhaps. But it may be hard to spot since it's normal for your weight to vary by as much as two pounds up or down through fluctuations in the amount of water it retains. And, just when it has started to fall, it may level off temporarily. Be patient.

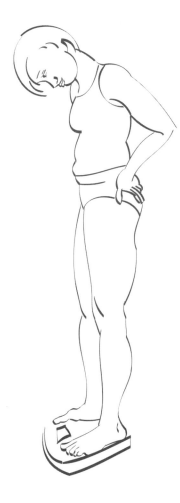

After all, you'll be losing around a pound a week from now until you reach the weight you want to reach.

So there's no need to overdo it. In fact, the more slowly and steadily you lose weight, the easier it may be to keep it off.

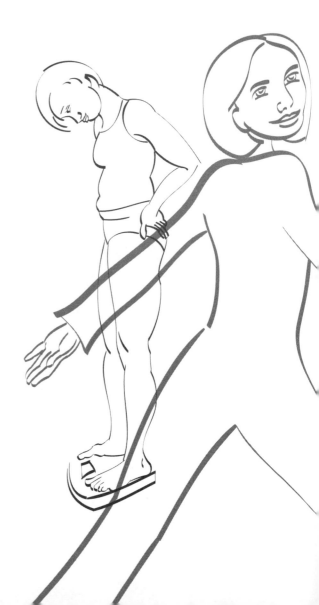

Pause point

To get the most from this book, you should pause after reading this page.

There's much more to come—but be sure to stop here and return to the book a few days later. Here's why.

In the days after you learn something new, your memory fades. You may forget most of what you learned. That might seem annoying, but if you remembered everything you had seen only once, your memory would quickly get overcrowded.

So how do you prevent fading? You need to reinforce what you want to remember. The best way to reinforce knowledge is simple: use it. That's why we recommend comparing the calories on food labels over the next few days or, better, making some substitutions to eliminate 500 calories a day.

Then come back to *Stikky Weight Management* and start at Sequence Two on the page after this one.

(We have noticed that, when readers continue straight on to Sequence Two, they often get stuck and don't complete it, or find that they forget what they have learned more quickly.)

If you are away from the book for more than a week, or if you don't get a chance to practice in between, you will want to review the end of Sequence One before starting Sequence Two.

When you're ready to continue, read from the next page to the **Pause point** at the end of Sequence Two on page 193.

And remember your promise: when asked a question in the text you will not flip ahead without attempting to answer it.

Sequence Two

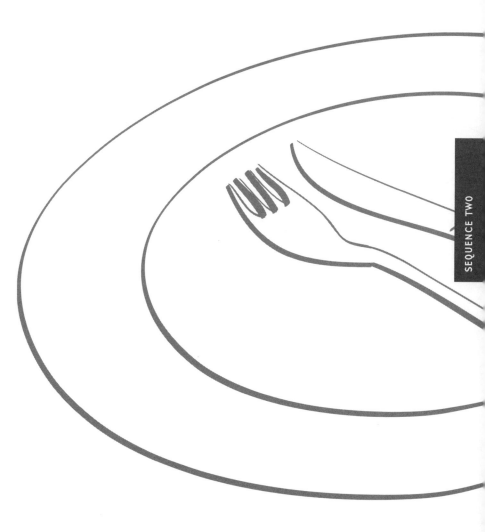

SEQUENCE TWO

Included in this sequence: America's top 10 food sources of calories, four good foods and three bad, surprising news about exercise, and the diet study with results so extraordinary it had to be stopped.

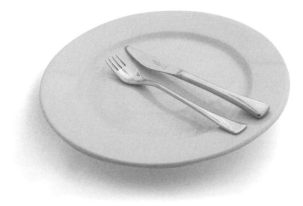

But first a brief recap.

How many calories in this candy bar? (Hint: it's the same as most other candy bars.)

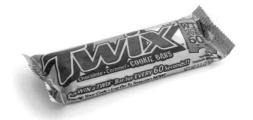

250.

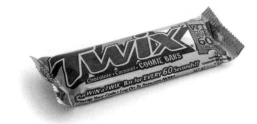

How many in an orange?

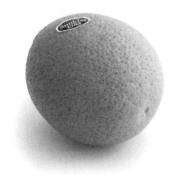

50.

Fruit is low in calories because it is 80% water. It helps fill you up for minimal calories (pretty much the opposite of a Twix).

Other classic high-in-water foods are soup and salad. But don't try living on just soup or salad as some diets recommend
—you'll go nuts.

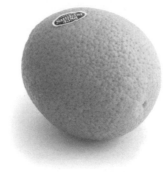

How many calories a day do you need to save in order to lose one pound a week?

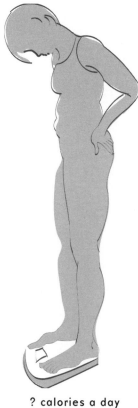

? calories a day
= 1 pound a week

500.

Here's an interesting fact: if you cut 2,000 calories a day —the maximum most people could cut without starving —you would lose 4 pounds a week (2,000 = 4 x 500).

So, anyone who says you can lose more than 4 pounds a week with their diet method can only be talking about surgery!

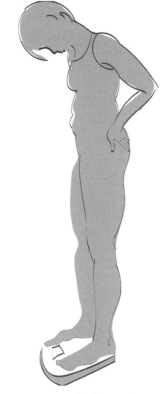

500 calories a day = 1 pound a week

If you made some substitutions after reading Sequence One, you may already have seen the results on your scale. If not, don't worry, it usually takes longer than a week.

Now you may be thinking, "Hold on. Changing what I eat is one thing, but don't I have to do lots of exercise too?"

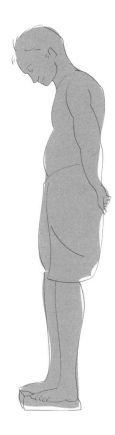

Exercise certainly helps, but not as much as you think.

If you read a book for an hour, you burn 75 calories. If instead you spend an hour working out at the gym (or some other vigorous exercise) you may burn as many as 500 calories more.

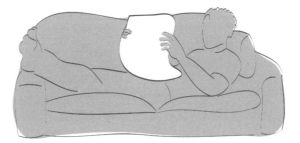

Sounds good, but…

…as you know by now, 500 calories a day is what you need to save each day to lose a pound a week.

To achieve this you would have to work out vigorously for an hour every single day, the equivalent of running 35 miles every week.

For most people, that's just not realistic.

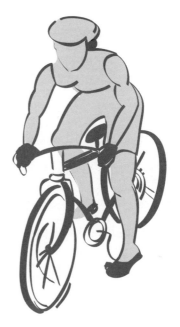

And, if you drink a sports drink during your workout or reward yourself afterwards with a slice of pizza, you put back most of the calories you burned.

People who do this can exercise regularly for months and lose little or nothing. It's much easier to eat 500 calories than to burn 500 calories.

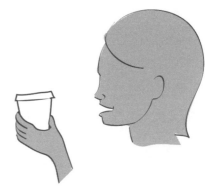

Being fit is still a good thing, of course, but how fit do you need to be?

Researchers looking into this question shocked everyone —including themselves—in the early 1990s when they found the answer: you can get most of the health benefits from exercise by *being just a bit fit*. People who are super-fit get little extra benefit.

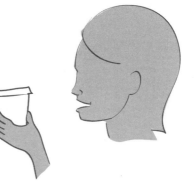

The researchers also uncovered a far better and easier way to get the benefits of exercise.

It doesn't cost anything. It doesn't involve any special equipment. It takes almost no time. And it isn't a recent fad —in fact, your distant ancestors got their exercise this way too.

It's…

Walking.

Studies have shown that even *30 minutes of brisk walking five times a week* can deliver all the benefits of structured exercise: improving your cardiovascular health (a good thing whatever your weight), lifting your mood, reducing stress, and burning some extra calories.

(So it's especially helpful when you have succeeded in losing weight and want to keep it off.)

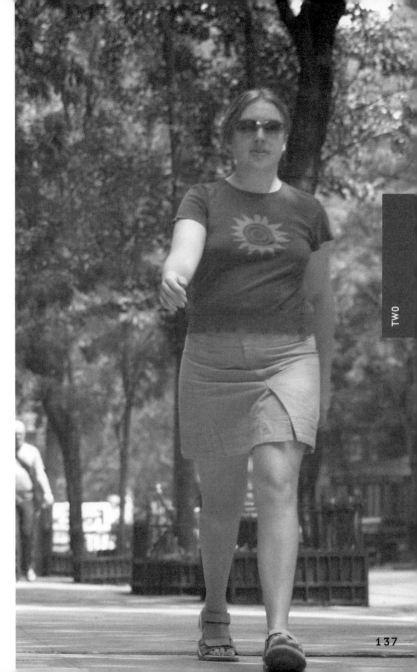

To count, it has to be *brisk* walking—the speed you walk when you're late for an appointment. Sauntering along isn't good enough.

You don't need to raise a sweat or be out of breath (though there's no harm in either, unless you have a heart condition).

Maybe you already do this much exercise; it's not so much. But two-thirds of Americans don't.

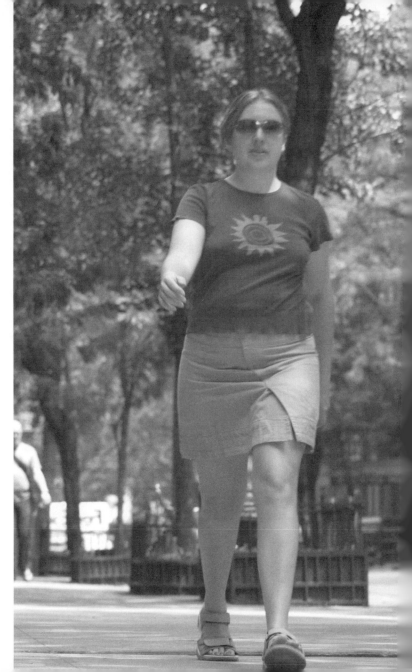

Most people have several opportunities every day to walk a little further.

For instance, picture yourself driving to the mall. Where might you park to improve your fitness?

Think about it and decide on your answer before flipping the page.

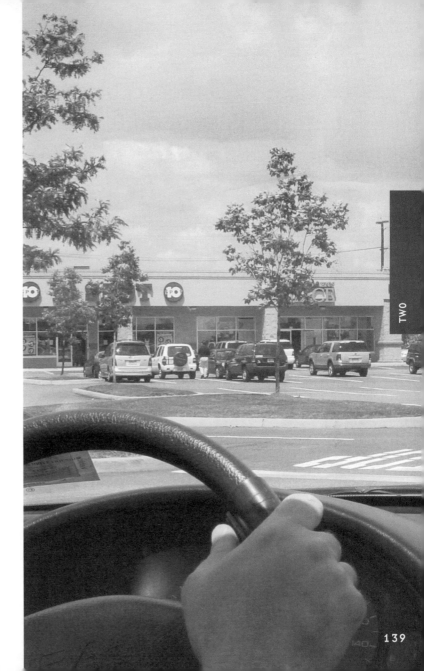

If you park in the far corner of the lot and walk briskly, that contributes to your 30 minutes a day.

(Plus, it's easier to find a parking space).

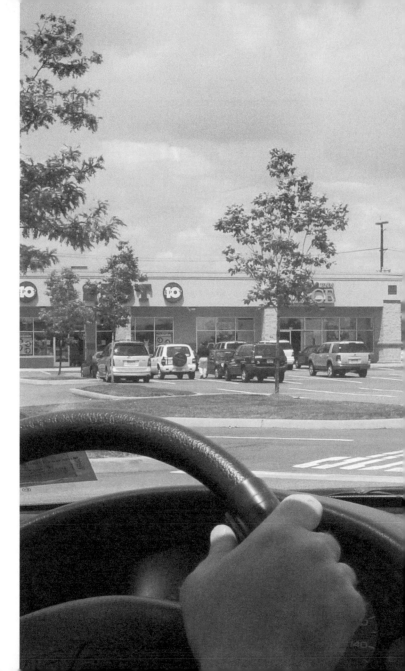

You have three items to take upstairs. What could you do to improve your fitness?

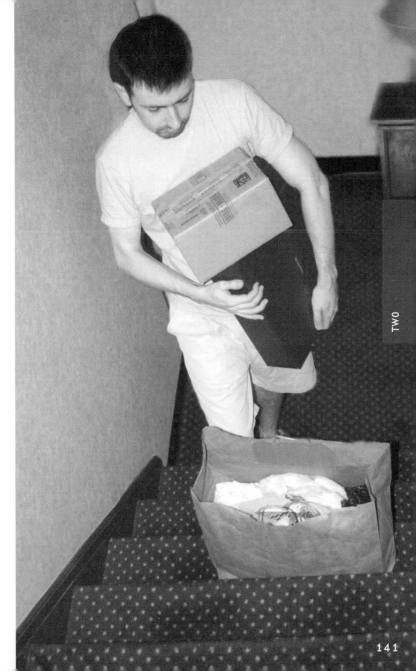

Take them up one at a time.

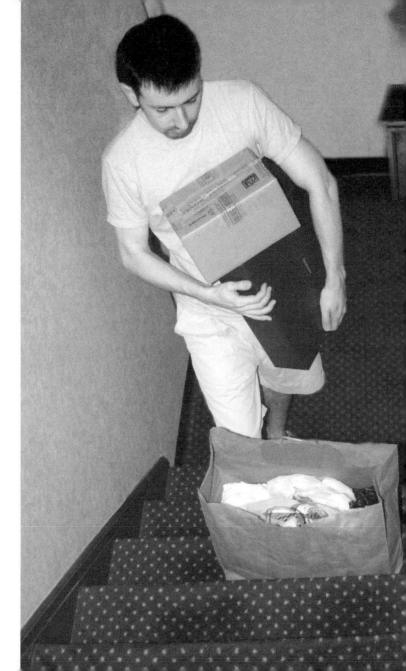

You are about to drive to a
local store for a few items,
what could you do to improve
your fitness?

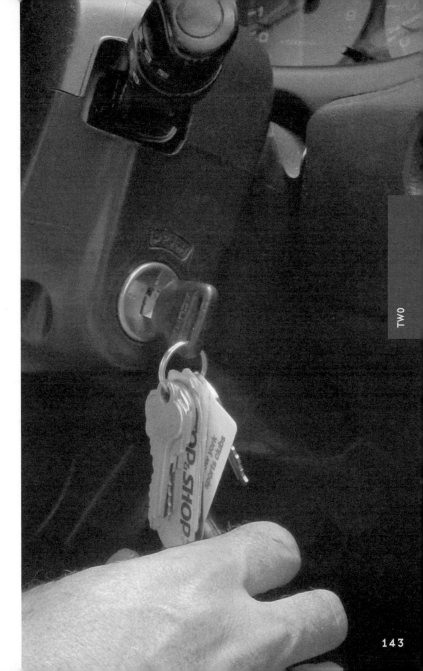

Leave the car and walk instead.

These revelations about diet and exercise are quite recent. In fact, scientists are only now discovering the truth about what is good or bad for you. (So what your mother told you may be out-of-date.)

Take, for example, a famous study begun in 1988 in Lyon, France. 605 heart attack survivors, men and women, were divided into two groups...

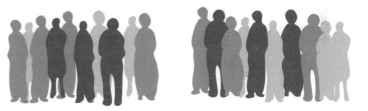

One group was given no specific dietary advice.

The other group followed a diet similar to that of Mediterraneans —eating the same amount of total fat as a typical diet, but replacing bad 'saturated' fat (like the fat in butter) with good 'unsaturated' fat (like that in olive oil).

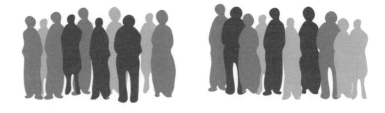

The researchers set things up this way since they had noticed that people in Mediterranean countries have fewer heart attacks.

But they were not prepared for what happened next.

Half-way through the study their ethics committee ordered them to stop it. The group following a Mediterranean diet had 60% fewer deaths so it was considered unethical not to tell the other group and let them switch diets.

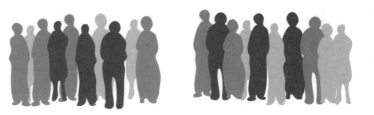

This study, and several others since, show that not all fat is bad fat.

Everyone knows cholesterol is bad—the less you eat the better.

Saturated fat is also bad. It's a proven clogger of arteries and cause of heart disease.

Now, when you check Nutrition Facts labels, you can ignore the total fat part and look for cholesterol and sat fat.
The lower the better.

Nutrition Facts
Serving Size 1 oz (28g/About 20 chips)
Servings Per Container About 6

Amount Per Serving

Calories 150	Calories from Fat 90

	% Daily Value*
Total Fat 10g	**15%**
Saturated Fat 3g	**15%**
Cholesterol 0mg	**0%**
Sodium 180mg	**8%**
Total Carbohydrate 15g	**5%**
Dietary Fiber 1g	**4%**
Sugars 0g	
Protein 2g	

Vitamin A 0%	•	Vitamin C 10%
Calcuim 0%	•	Iron 0%

* Percent Daily Values are based on a 2,000 calorie diet.
  Your daily values may be higher or lower depending
  on your calorie needs:

	Calories:	2,000	2,500
Total Fat	Less than	65g	80g
Sat Fat	Less than	20g	25g
Cholesterol	Less than	300mg	300mg
Sodium	Less than	2,400mg	2,400mg
Total Carbohydrate		300g	375g
Dietary Fiber		25g	30g

Calories per gram: Fat 9 • Carbohydrate 4 • Protein 4

TWO

So which of these two is better
for you?

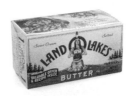

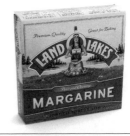

Nutrition Facts

Serving Size 1 Tbsp (14g)
Servings Per Container 32

Amount Per Serving

Calories 100	Calories from Fat 100
	% Daily Value*
Total Fat 11g	**17**%
Saturated Fat 8g	**38**%
Cholesterol 30mg	**10**%
Sodium 85mg	**4**%
Total Carbohydrate 0g	**0**%
Protein 0g	

Vitamin A 8%

Not a significant source of dietary fiber, sugars,
vitamin C, calcium, and iron.

* Percent Daily Values are based on a 2,000 calorie diet.

Nutrition Facts

Serving Size 1 Tbsp (14g)
Servings Per Container 32

Amount Per Serving

Calories 100	Calories from Fat 100
	% Daily Value*
Total Fat 11g	**17**%
Saturated Fat 2g	**11**%
Polyunsaturated Fat 3.5g	
Monounsaturated Fat 3g	
Cholesterol 0mg	**0**%
Sodium 115mg	**5**%
Total Carbohydrate 0g	**0**%
Protein 0g	

Vitamin A 10%

Not a significant source of dietary fiber, sugars,
vitamin C, calcium, and iron.

* Percent Daily Values are based on a 2,000 calorie diet.

The margarine. It has the same number of calories, same amount of total fat, but no cholesterol and much less sat fat.

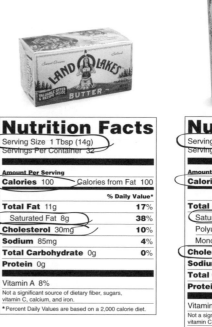

Nutrition Facts

Serving Size 1 Tbsp (14g)
Servings Per Container 32

Amount Per Serving

Calories 100   Calories from Fat 100

	% Daily Value*
Total Fat 11g	17%
Saturated Fat 8g	38%
Cholesterol 30mg	10%
Sodium 85mg	4%
Total Carbohydrate 0g	0%
Protein 0g	

Vitamin A 8%

Not a significant source of dietary fiber, sugars, vitamin C, calcium, and iron.

* Percent Daily Values are based on a 2,000 calorie diet.

Nutrition Facts

Serving Size 1 Tbsp (14g)
Servings Per Container 32

Amount Per Serving

Calories 100   Calories from Fat 100

	% Daily Value*
Total Fat 11g	17%
Saturated Fat 2g	11%
Polyunsaturated Fat 3.5g	
Monounsaturated Fat 3g	
Cholesterol 0mg	0%
Sodium 115mg	5%
Total Carbohydrate 0g	0%
Protein 0g	

Vitamin A 10%

Not a significant source of dietary fiber, sugars, vitamin C, calcium, and iron.

* Percent Daily Values are based on a 2,000 calorie diet.

Now compare the margarine to olive oil. Which is better for you?

(Forget what you think the answer should be, check the labels and find out the truth.)

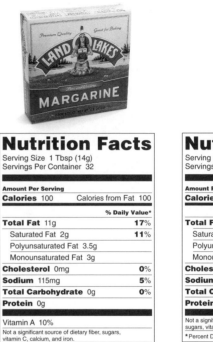

Nutrition Facts

Serving Size 1 Tbsp (14g)
Servings Per Container 32

Amount Per Serving		
Calories 100	Calories from Fat 100	
		% Daily Value*
Total Fat 11g		**17**%
Saturated Fat 2g		**11**%
Polyunsaturated Fat 3.5g		
Monounsaturated Fat 3g		
Cholesterol 0mg		**0**%
Sodium 115mg		**5**%
Total Carbohydrate 0g		**0**%
Protein 0g		

Vitamin A 10%

Not a significant source of dietary fiber, sugars, vitamin C, calcium, and iron.

* Percent Daily Values are based on a 2,000 calorie diet.

Nutrition Facts

Serving Size 1 Tbsp (15ml)
Servings Per Container 33

Amount Per Serving		
Calories 120	Calories from Fat 120	
		% Daily Value*
Total Fat 14g		**22**%
Saturated Fat 2g		**10**%
Polyunsaturated Fat 2g		
Monounsaturated Fat 10g		
Cholesterol 0mg		**0**%
Sodium 0mg		**0**%
Total Carbohydrate 0g		**0**%
Protein 0g		

Not a significant source of cholesterol, dietary fiber, sugars, vitamin A, vitamin C, calcium, and iron.

* Percent Daily Values are based on a 2,000 calorie diet.

TWO

They both have low sat fat and no cholesterol, though this margarine, unexpectedly, has slightly fewer calories than the olive oil. (But be careful: margarines vary widely.)

Good fat (like olive oil in the Mediterranean diet and the soybean oil in this margarine) helps you feel full. Which is why people who avoid fat altogether have a tough time sticking to their diet.

Nutrition Facts
Serving Size 1 Tbsp (14g)
Servings Per Container 32

Amount Per Serving

Calories 100   Calories from Fat 100

                                  % Daily Value*

Total Fat 11g	17%
Saturated Fat 2g	11%
Polyunsaturated Fat 3.5g	
Monounsaturated Fat 3g	
Cholesterol 0mg	0%
Sodium 115mg	5%
Total Carbohydrate 0g	0%
Protein 0g	

Vitamin A 10%

Not a significant source of dietary fiber, sugars, vitamin C, calcium, and iron.

* Percent Daily Values are based on a 2,000 calorie diet.

Nutrition Facts
Serving Size 1 Tbsp (15ml)
Servings Per Container 33

Amount Per Serving

Calories 120   Calories from Fat 120

                                  % Daily Value*

Total Fat 14g	22%
Saturated Fat 2g	10%
Polyunsaturated Fat 2g	
Monounsaturated Fat 10g	
Cholesterol 0mg	0%
Sodium 0mg	0%
Total Carbohydrate 0g	0%
Protein 0g	

Not a significant source of cholesterol, dietary fiber, sugars, vitamin A, vitamin C, calcium, and iron.

* Percent Daily Values are based on a 2,000 calorie diet.

What about these two?

The muffin on the left is a
Dunkin Donuts Blueberry Muffin.
The one on the right is their
Reduced Fat Blueberry Muffin.

Which would you choose?

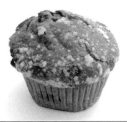
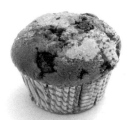

Nutrition Facts

Serving Size 1 muffin
Servings Per Container 1

Amount Per Serving

Calories 490   Calories from Fat 160

	% Daily Value*
Total Fat 18g	**30%**
Saturated Fat 6g	**30%**
Cholesterol 75mg	**25%**
Sodium 630mg	**25%**
Total Carbohydrate 75g	**25%**
Dietary Fiber 2g	**8%**
Sugars 39g	
Protein 8g	

Vitamin A 4%	•	Vitamin C 0%
Calcuim 6%	•	Iron 15%

*Percent Daily Values are based on a 2,000 calorie diet.
Your daily values may be higher or lower depending
on your calorie needs:

		Calories:	2,000	2,500
Total Fat	Less than		65g	80g
Sat Fat	Less than		20g	25g
Cholesterol	Less than		300mg	300mg
Sodium	Less than		2,400mg	2,400mg
Total Carbohydrate			300g	375g
Dietary Fiber			25g	30g

Calories per gram: Fat 9 • Carbohydrate 4 • Protein 4

Nutrition Facts

Serving Size 1 muffin
Servings Per Container 1

Amount Per Serving

Calories 450   Calories from Fat 120

	% Daily Value*
Total Fat 13g	**20%**
Saturated Fat 3.5g	**20%**
Cholesterol 70mg	**25%**
Sodium 650mg	**25%**
Total Carbohydrate 74g	**25%**
Dietary Fiber 2g	**8%**
Sugars 35g	
Protein 9g	

Vitamin A 2%	•	Vitamin C 0%
Calcuim 8%	•	Iron 15%

*Percent Daily Values are based on a 2,000 calorie diet.
Your daily values may be higher or lower depending
on your calorie needs:

		Calories:	2,000	2,500
Total Fat	Less than		65g	80g
Sat Fat	Less than		20g	25g
Cholesterol	Less than		300mg	300mg
Sodium	Less than		2,400mg	2,400mg
Total Carbohydrate			300g	375g
Dietary Fiber			25g	30g

Calories per gram: Fat 9 • Carbohydrate 4 • Protein 4

The reduced fat muffin has less sat fat and cholesterol but both have a huge number of calories—nearly 500.

So hopefully you wouldn't choose either one. 'Reduced fat' does not always mean 'healthy'.

You may not have heard much about sat fat before. It's worth knowing more about which foods contain it...

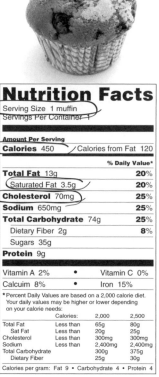

Nutrition Facts

Serving Size 1 muffin
Servings Per Container 1

Amount Per Serving

Calories 490   Calories from Fat 160

	% Daily Value*
Total Fat 18g	**30%**
Saturated Fat 6g	**30%**
Cholesterol 75mg	**25%**
Sodium 630mg	**25%**
Total Carbohydrate 75g	**25%**
Dietary Fiber 2g	**8%**
Sugars 39g	
Protein 8g	

Vitamin A 4%	•	Vitamin C 0%
Calcuim 6%	•	Iron 15%

*Percent Daily Values are based on a 2,000 calorie diet. Your daily values may be higher or lower depending on your calorie needs:

		Calories:	2,000	2,500
Total Fat	Less than		65g	80g
Sat Fat	Less than		20g	25g
Cholesterol	Less than		300mg	300mg
Sodium	Less than		2,400mg	2,400mg
Total Carbohydrate			300g	375g
Dietary Fiber			25g	30g

Calories per gram: Fat 9 • Carbohydrate 4 • Protein 4

Nutrition Facts

Serving Size 1 muffin
Servings Per Container 1

Amount Per Serving

Calories 450   Calories from Fat 120

	% Daily Value*
Total Fat 13g	**20%**
Saturated Fat 3.5g	**20%**
Cholesterol 70mg	**25%**
Sodium 650mg	**25%**
Total Carbohydrate 74g	**25%**
Dietary Fiber 2g	**8%**
Sugars 35g	
Protein 9g	

Vitamin A 2%	•	Vitamin C 0%
Calcuim 8%	•	Iron 15%

*Percent Daily Values are based on a 2,000 calorie diet. Your daily values may be higher or lower depending on your calorie needs:

		Calories:	2,000	2,500
Total Fat	Less than		65g	80g
Sat Fat	Less than		20g	25g
Cholesterol	Less than		300mg	300mg
Sodium	Less than		2,400mg	2,400mg
Total Carbohydrate			300g	375g
Dietary Fiber			25g	30g

Calories per gram: Fat 9 • Carbohydrate 4 • Protein 4

TWO

Margarine, butter and cakes contribute a high proportion of the sat fat in our diet, but they are not the worst culprits as you can see.

What food do you think is the single biggest contributor of sat fat in the American diet?
Take a guess.

1	?	12.7%
2	Beef	12.4%
3	Milk	10.5%
4	Cakes, cookies, quick breads, doughnuts	5.0%
5	Margarine	4.8%
6	Butter	4.1%

TWO

Cheese is the #1 contributor of saturated fat in US diets.

A quick look at some labels will reveal how to minimize the sat fat you get from cheese…

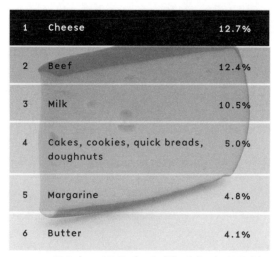

1	Cheese	12.7%
2	Beef	12.4%
3	Milk	10.5%
4	Cakes, cookies, quick breads, doughnuts	5.0%
5	Margarine	4.8%
6	Butter	4.1%

SOURCE: AF Subar, SM Krebs-Smith, A Cook, LL Kahle 'Dietary sources of nutrients among US adults, 1989 to 1991' *Journal of the American Dietetic Association*, May 1998

Here are two types of cheese: a 16-ounce tub of cottage cheese and a bar of Cheddar. You can see which is lower sat fat at a glance.

Now, if you substitute 4 ounces of cottage cheese (1 serving) for 2 ounces of Cheddar, how many calories do you save?

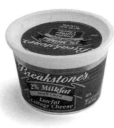

Nutrition Facts

Serving Size 1/2 cup (4 oz)
Servings Per Container About 4

Amount Per Serving

Calories 90	Calories from Fat 20

	% Daily Value*
Total Fat 2.5g	**4%**
Saturated Fat 1.5g	**8%**
Cholesterol 15mg	**5%**
Sodium 400mg	**17%**
Total Carbohydrate 6g	**2%**
Fiber 0g	**0%**
Sugars 4g	
Protein 12g	**24%**

Vitamin A 4%	•	Vitamin C 0%
Calcuim 8%	•	Iron 0%

*Percent Daily Values are based on a 2,000 calorie diet.

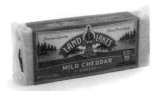

Nutrition Facts

Serving Size 1 oz
(28g/about a 1-inch cube)
Servings 8
Calories 110
Fat Cal. 80
*Percent Daily Values (DV) are based on a 2,000 calorie diet.

Amount/Serving	%DV*	Amount/Serving	%DV*
Total Fat 9g	**14%**	**Total Carb.** less than 1g	**0%**
Sat Fat 6g	**30%**	Fiber 0g	**0%**
Cholest. 30mg	**10%**	Sugars 0g	
Sodium 180mg	**7%**	**Protein** 7g	

Vitamin A 8% • Vitamin C 0% • Calcium 20% • Iron 0%

2 ounces of Cheddar is
2 x 110 = 220 calories.
4 ounces of cottage cheese is
90 calories.

So you save a full 130 calories.

(Here's another idea: in salads
with cheese, substitute a smaller
amount of a more strongly
flavored cheese like Parmesan or
Sharp Cheddar.)

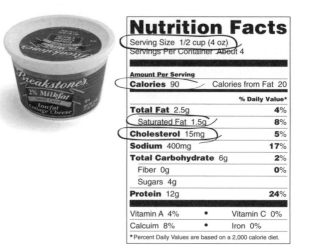

Nutrition Facts	
Serving Size 1/2 cup (4 oz)	
Servings Per Container About 4	
Amount Per Serving	
Calories 90	Calories from Fat 20
	% Daily Value*
Total Fat 2.5g	4%
Saturated Fat 1.5g	8%
Cholesterol 15mg	5%
Sodium 400mg	17%
Total Carbohydrate 6g	2%
Fiber 0g	0%
Sugars 4g	
Protein 12g	24%
Vitamin A 4% • Vitamin C 0%	
Calcuim 8% • Iron 0%	
*Percent Daily Values are based on a 2,000 calorie diet.	

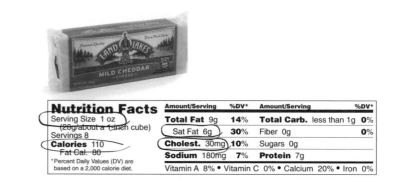

Nutrition Facts	Amount/Serving	%DV*	Amount/Serving	%DV*
Serving Size 1 oz (28g/about a 1-inch cube) Servings 8	**Total Fat** 9g	**14%**	**Total Carb.** less than 1g	**0%**
	Sat Fat 6g	**30%**	Fiber 0g	**0%**
Calories 110 Fat Cal. 80	**Cholest.** 30mg	**10%**	Sugars 0g	
	Sodium 180mg	**7%**	**Protein** 7g	
*Percent Daily Values (DV) are based on a 2,000 calorie diet.	Vitamin A 8% • Vitamin C 0% • Calcium 20% • Iron 0%			

Beef is the #2 contributor of sat fat.

If you want to cut down on sat fat, now is a good time to make a commitment. Choose one of these instead: extra-lean beef, or pork tenderloin, or chicken (without the skin, which can contain about as much fat as the rest of the breast).

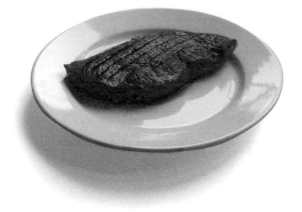

(You made a commitment, right?)

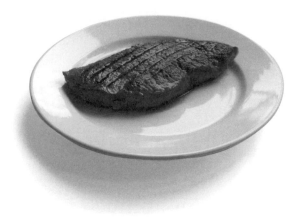

Milk is the #3 contributor of sat fat.

Switching to non-fat or 1% milk reduces sat fat as well as saving you calories. Remember how many calories you save by choosing non-fat milk in a grande latte?

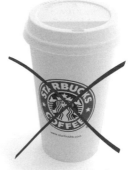

Whole milk grande latte

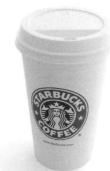

Non-fat grande latte
save ? calories

100.

(150 if you also substitute tall
for grande.)

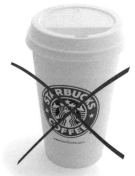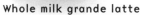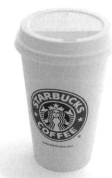

Whole milk grande latte   Non-fat grande latte
                                 save 100 calories

TWO

Sat fat is bad fat, but there is worse—trans fat.

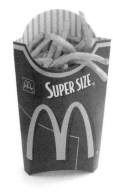

Trans fat is a sort of man-made, concentrated sat fat that helps increase shelf life.

Sounds bad? It is. The Institute of Medicine says trans fats have "no known benefit to human health" and are directly linked to heart disease.

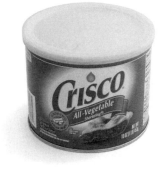

Deep-fried foods or foods that list 'hydrogenated' ingredients are most likely to include trans fat.

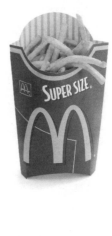

(So the scene in Woody Allen's *Sleeper* when future scientists discover that steak and deep-fried food are the key to healthy living is unfortunately not going to come true.)

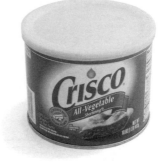

To make things easier, the FDA recently decreed that trans fat must be listed on Nutrition Facts labels from 2006.

Until then, just avoid foods that list 'hydrogenated' or 'partially hydrogenated' ingredients.

The margarine we looked at earlier is an example—here are the ingredients listed on its label. (So olive oil was a better choice after all.)

Nutrition Facts

Serving Size 1 cup (228g)
Servings Per Container 2

Amount Per Serving

Calories 260	Calories from Fat 120

	% Daily Value*
Total Fat 13g	20%
Saturated Fat 5g	25%
Trans Fat 2g	
Cholesterol 30mg	10%
Sodium 660mg	28%
Total Carbohydrate 31g	10%

INGREDIENTS: LIQUID SOYBEAN OIL, PARTIALLY HYDROGENATED SOYBEAN OIL, WATER, BUTTERMILK, SALT, SOY LECITHIN, SODIUM BENZOATE (AS A PRESERVATIVE), VEGETABLE MONO AND DIGLYCERIDES, ARTIFICIAL FLAVOR, VITAMIN A PALMITATE, COLORED WITH BETA CAROTENE (PROVITAMIN A).

Cholesterol, sat fat, trans fat…that's enough about bad foods.

Let's turn to foods that do you good in their own right (not just by saving calories).

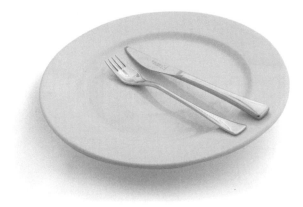

If you are looking, you'll probably see a press story every month announcing the discovery of a new 'miracle' food.

Beta carotene, soy, zinc, coral calcium, etc...

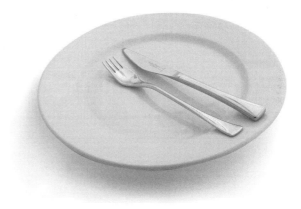

Some of these reports are
unproven; many are wishful
thinking. Now and then, the
benefits are real but only if you
consume enormous amounts of
one specific food, and even then
the effects may be weak.

In fact, after literally thousands
of major randomized trials,
there are only four foods that
experts agree you should eat
more of if you can.

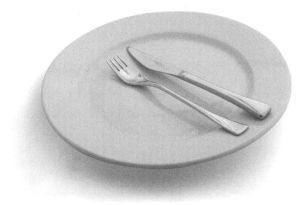

Eating fish once a week has been found to protect against stroke.

(Interestingly, eating fish more often than that does not seem to increase the protection.)

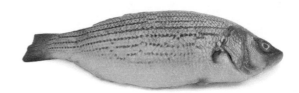

Fiber has been linked, in study after study, to a reduction in the risk of diabetes and heart disease.

The more you eat, the better.

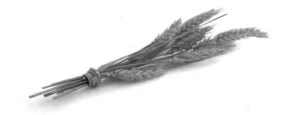

Here are the top contributors of
fiber to the American diet.

Would you like to guess the
missing item in the #1 spot?

1	?	14.6%
2	Ready-to-eat cereal	8.0%
3	Dried beans, lentils	7.9%
4	Potatoes (white)	7.3%
5	Tomatoes	5.7%
6	Pasta	4.3%

Bread.

1	Yeast bread	14.6%
2	Ready-to-eat cereal	8.0%
3	Dried beans, lentils	7.9%
4	Potatoes (white)	7.3%
5	Tomatoes	5.7%
6	Pasta	4.3%

SOURCE: AF Subar, SM Krebs-Smith, A Cook, LL Kahle 'Dietary sources of nutrients among US adults, 1989 to 1991' *Journal of the American Dietetic Association*, May 1998

But, as you know by now, foods in the same category can be quite different.

Which of these two breads is the better choice?

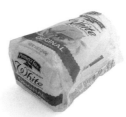

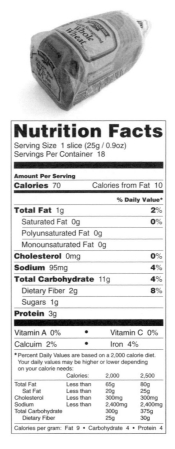

Nutrition Facts

Serving Size 1 slice (25g / 0.9oz)
Servings Per Container 18

Amount Per Serving

Calories 70	Calories from Fat 10
	% Daily Value*
Total Fat 1g	**2%**
Saturated Fat 0g	**0%**
Polyunsaturated Fat 0g	
Monounsaturated Fat 0g	
Cholesterol 0mg	**0%**
Sodium 95mg	**4%**
Total Carbohydrate 11g	**4%**
Dietary Fiber 2g	**8%**
Sugars 1g	
Protein 3g	

Vitamin A 0%	•	Vitamin C 0%
Calcuim 2%	•	Iron 4%

*Percent Daily Values are based on a 2,000 calorie diet.
Your daily values may be higher or lower depending
on your calorie needs:

	Calories:	2,000	2,500
Total Fat	Less than	65g	80g
Sat Fat	Less than	20g	25g
Cholesterol	Less than	300mg	300mg
Sodium	Less than	2,400mg	2,400mg
Total Carbohydrate		300g	375g
Dietary Fiber		25g	30g

Calories per gram: Fat 9 • Carbohydrate 4 • Protein 4

Nutrition Facts

Serving Size 1 slice (25g / 0.9oz)
Servings Per Container 18

Amount Per Serving

Calories 70	Calories from Fat 15
	% Daily Value*
Total Fat 1.5g	**2%**
Saturated Fat 0g	**0%**
Polyunsaturated Fat 0g	
Monounsaturated Fat 0.5g	
Cholesterol 0mg	**0%**
Sodium 135mg	**6%**
Total Carbohydrate 13g	**4%**
Dietary Fiber 0g	**0%**
Sugars 2g	
Protein 2g	

Vitamin A 0%	•	Vitamin C 0%
Calcium 2%	•	Iron 4%
Thiamin 6%	•	Riboflavin 4%
Niacin 4%	•	Folate 4%

*Percent Daily Values are based on a 2,000 calorie diet.
Your daily values may be higher or lower depending
on your calorie needs:

	Calories:	2,000	2,500
Total Fat	Less than	65g	80g
Sat Fat	Less than	20g	25g
Cholesterol	Less than	300mg	300mg
Sodium	Less than	2,400mg	2,400mg
Total Carbohydrate		300g	375g
Dietary Fiber		25g	30g

Calories per gram: Fat 9 • Carbohydrate 4 • Protein 4

The wholewheat bread has the same number of calories but more fiber, so is the better choice.

(So now you know all five interesting areas on a Nutrition Facts label.)

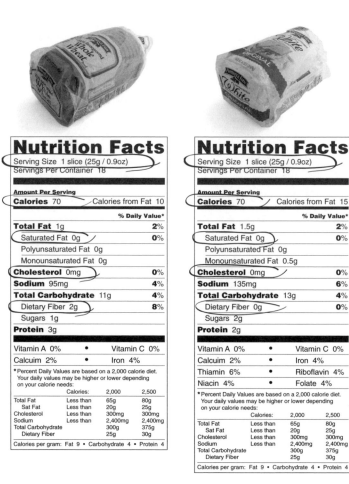

Nutrition Facts

Serving Size 1 slice (25g / 0.9oz)
Servings Per Container 18

Amount Per Serving

Calories 70   Calories from Fat 10

% Daily Value*

Total Fat 1g	2%
Saturated Fat 0g	0%
Polyunsaturated Fat 0g	
Monounsaturated Fat 0g	
Cholesterol 0mg	0%
Sodium 95mg	4%
Total Carbohydrate 11g	4%
Dietary Fiber 2g	8%
Sugars 1g	
Protein 3g	

Vitamin A 0%	•	Vitamin C 0%
Calcuim 2%	•	Iron 4%

*Percent Daily Values are based on a 2,000 calorie diet. Your daily values may be higher or lower depending on your calorie needs:

		Calories:	2,000	2,500
Total Fat	Less than		65g	80g
Sat Fat	Less than		20g	25g
Cholesterol	Less than		300mg	300mg
Sodium	Less than		2,400mg	2,400mg
Total Carbohydrate			300g	375g
Dietary Fiber			25g	30g

Calories per gram: Fat 9 • Carbohydrate 4 • Protein 4

Nutrition Facts

Serving Size 1 slice (25g / 0.9oz)
Servings Per Container 18

Amount Per Serving

Calories 70   Calories from Fat 15

% Daily Value*

Total Fat 1.5g	2%
Saturated Fat 0g	0%
Polyunsaturated Fat 0g	
Monounsaturated Fat 0.5g	
Cholesterol 0mg	0%
Sodium 135mg	6%
Total Carbohydrate 13g	4%
Dietary Fiber 0g	0%
Sugars 2g	
Protein 2g	

Vitamin A 0%	•	Vitamin C 0%
Calcuim 2%	•	Iron 4%
Thiamin 6%	•	Riboflavin 4%
Niacin 4%	•	Folate 4%

*Percent Daily Values are based on a 2,000 calorie diet. Your daily values may be higher or lower depending on your calorie needs:

		Calories:	2,000	2,500
Total Fat	Less than		65g	80g
Sat Fat	Less than		20g	25g
Cholesterol	Less than		300mg	300mg
Sodium	Less than		2,400mg	2,400mg
Total Carbohydrate			300g	375g
Dietary Fiber			25g	30g

Calories per gram: Fat 9 • Carbohydrate 4 • Protein 4

Which of these two cereals is better for you?

(Cereal labels are the most complex, so this may take you a little longer to figure out.)

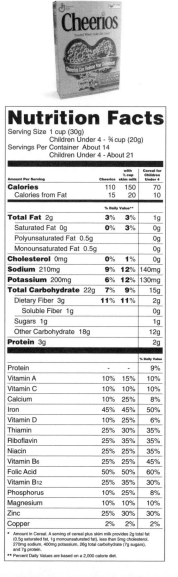

Nutrition Facts

Serving Size 1 cup (30g)
Children Under 4 - ¾ cup (20g)
Servings Per Container About 14
Children Under 4 - About 21

Amount Per Serving	Cheerios	with ½ cup skim milk	Cereal for Children Under 4
Calories	110	150	70
Calories from Fat	15	20	10
	% Daily Value**		
Total Fat 2g	**3%**	**3%**	1g
Saturated Fat 0g	**0%**	**3%**	0g
Polyunsaturated Fat 0.5g			0g
Monounsaturated Fat 0.5g			0g
Cholesterol 0mg	**0%**	**1%**	0g
Sodium 210mg	**9%**	**12%**	140mg
Potassium 200mg	**6%**	**12%**	130mg
Total Carbohydrate 22g	**7%**	**9%**	15g
Dietary Fiber 3g	**11%**	**11%**	2g
Soluble Fiber 1g			0g
Sugars 1g			1g
Other Carbohydrate 18g			12g
Protein 3g			2g
	% Daily Value		
Protein	-	-	9%
Vitamin A	10%	15%	10%
Vitamin C	10%	10%	10%
Calcium	10%	25%	8%
Iron	45%	45%	50%
Vitamin D	10%	25%	6%
Thiamin	25%	30%	35%
Riboflavin	25%	35%	35%
Niacin	25%	25%	35%
Vitamin B6	25%	25%	45%
Folic Acid	50%	50%	60%
Vitamin B12	25%	35%	30%
Phosphorus	10%	25%	8%
Magnesium	10%	10%	10%
Zinc	25%	30%	30%
Copper	2%	2%	2%

*   Amount in Cereal. A serving of cereal plus skim milk provides 2g total fat (0.5g saturated fat, 1g monounsaturated fat), less than 5mg cholesterol, 270mg sodium, 400mg potassium, 26g total carbohydrate (7g sugars), and 7g protein.
**   Percent Daily Values are based on a 2,000 calorie diet.

Nutrition Facts

Serving Size 1/2 cup (31g/1.1oz)
Servings Per Container About 17

Amount Per Serving	Cereal	Cereal with ½ cup Vitamins A&D Fat Free Milk
Calories	80	120
Calories from Fat	10	10
	% Daily Value**	
Total Fat 1g*	**2%**	**2%**
Saturated Fat 0g	**0%**	**0%**
Cholesterol 0mg	**0%**	**0%**
Sodium 80mg	**3%**	**6%**
Potassium 350mg	**10%**	**16%**
Total Carbohydrate 23g	**8%**	**10%**
Dietary Fiber 10g	**40%**	**40%**
Soluble Fiber 1g		
Sugars 6g		
Other Carbohydrate 7g		
Protein 4g		
Vitamin A	10%	15%
Vitamin C	10%	10%
Calcium	10%	25%
Iron	25%	25%
Vitamin D	10%	25%
Thiamin	25%	30%
Riboflavin	25%	35%
Niacin	25%	25%
Vitamin B6	100%	100%
Folic Acid	100%	100%
Vitamin B12	100%	110%
Phosphorus	35%	45%
Magnesium	25%	30%
Zinc	10%	15%
Copper	10%	10%

*   Amount in cereal. One half cup of fat free milk contributes an additional 40 calories, 65mg sodium, 6g total carbohydrate (6g sugars), and 4g protein.
**   Percent Daily Values are based on a 2,000 calorie diet.

All-Bran has fewer calories and more fiber—but that's only for half a cup.

So replacing a whole cup of Cheerios with half a cup of All-Bran is a good substitution; but not if you replace it with a whole cup of All-Bran (which most people would, naturally).

It pays to read the label closely.

Nutrition Facts (Cheerios)

Serving Size 1 cup (30g)
Children Under 4 - ¾ cup (20g)
Servings Per Container About 14
Children Under 4 - About 21

Amount Per Serving	Cheerios	with ½ cup skim milk	Cereal for Children Under 4
Calories	110	150	70
Calories from Fat	15	20	10

	% Daily Value**		
Total Fat 2g	3%	3%	1g
Saturated Fat 0g	0%	3%	0g
Polyunsaturated Fat 0.5g			0g
Monounsaturated Fat 0.5g			0g
Cholesterol 0mg	0%	1%	0g
Sodium 210mg	9%	12%	140mg
Potassium 200mg	6%	12%	130mg
Total Carbohydrate 22g	7%	9%	15g
Dietary Fiber 3g	11%	11%	2g
Soluble Fiber 1g			0g
Sugars 1g			1g
Other Carbohydrate 18g			12g
Protein 3g			2g

			% Daily Value
Protein	-	-	9%
Vitamin A	10%	15%	10%
Vitamin C	10%	10%	10%
Calcium	10%	25%	8%
Iron	45%	45%	50%
Vitamin D	10%	25%	6%
Thiamin	25%	30%	35%
Riboflavin	25%	35%	35%
Niacin	25%	25%	35%
Vitamin B6	25%	25%	45%
Folic Acid	50%	50%	60%
Vitamin B12	25%	35%	30%
Phosphorus	10%	25%	8%
Magnesium	10%	10%	10%
Zinc	25%	30%	30%
Copper	2%	2%	2%

* Amount in Cereal. A serving of cereal plus skim milk provides 2g total fat (0.5g saturated fat, 1g monounsaturated fat), less than 5mg cholesterol, 270mg sodium, 400mg potassium, 26g total carbohydrate (7g sugars), and 7g protein.
** Percent Daily Values are based on a 2,000 calorie diet.

Nutrition Facts (All-Bran)

Serving Size 1/2 cup (31g/1.1oz)
Servings Per Container About 17

Amount Per Serving	Cereal	Cereal with ½ cup Vitamins A&D Fat Free Milk
Calories	80	120
Calories from Fat	10	10

	% Daily Value**	
Total Fat 1g*	2%	2%
Saturated Fat 0g	0%	0%
Cholesterol 0mg	0%	0%
Sodium 80mg	3%	6%
Potassium 350mg	10%	16%
Total Carbohydrate 23g	8%	10%
Dietary Fiber 10g	40%	40%
Soluble Fiber 1g		
Sugars 6g		
Other Carbohydrate 7g		
Protein 4g		

Vitamin A	10%	15%
Vitamin C	10%	10%
Calcium	10%	25%
Iron	25%	25%
Vitamin D	10%	25%
Thiamin	25%	30%
Riboflavin	25%	35%
Niacin	25%	25%
Vitamin B6	100%	100%
Folic Acid	100%	100%
Vitamin B12	100%	110%
Phosphorus	35%	45%
Magnesium	25%	30%
Zinc	10%	15%
Copper	10%	10%

* Amount in cereal. One half cup of fat free milk contributes an additional 40 calories, 65mg sodium, 6g total carbohydrate (6g sugars), and 4g protein.
** Percent Daily Values are based on a 2,000 calorie diet.

So, fish, fiber…what else? Fruit and vegetables have been found to reduce the risk of just about everything—stroke, cancer, hypertension, cataracts. Again, the more you eat, the better.

Here are America's favorite fruit and vegetables; some may surprise you.

For fun, guess the #1 fruit and the #1 vegetable.

1	?	13.9%
2	Apple	10.3%
3	Orange	4.8%
4	Grape	3.3%
5	Cantaloupe	3.3%
6	Strawberry	2.6%

1	?	15.6%
2	Lettuce	10.3%
3	Tomato	8.8%
4	Mustard	4.6%
5	Cucumber, cucumber pickles	4.5%
6	Onions	4.5%

(These figures exclude juices, by the way. If they were included, orange juice would win by a long way.)

Potatoes pack the calories in. A 3" x 4" spud is 150 calories, the same as a Bud. A tomato that weighs the same is just 50 calories.

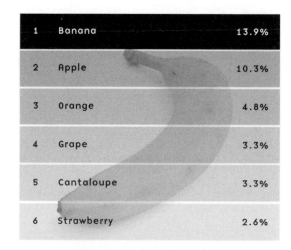

1	Banana	13.9%
2	Apple	10.3%
3	Orange	4.8%
4	Grape	3.3%
5	Cantaloupe	3.3%
6	Strawberry	2.6%

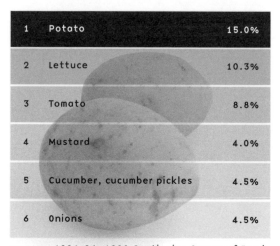

1	Potato	15.0%
2	Lettuce	10.3%
3	Tomato	8.8%
4	Mustard	4.0%
5	Cucumber, cucumber pickles	4.5%
6	Onions	4.5%

SOURCE: *1994-96, 1998 Continuing Survey of Food Intakes by Individuals*, USDA, www.barc.usda.gov/foodsurvey/home.htm

What about vitamins? Most Americans get the vitamins they need with the exception of one: folic acid (also known as folate), which has been shown to reduce the risk of heart disease.

You can get folic acid from a fortified breakfast cereal or from lentils, spinach, or pasta. If you don't eat much of these, and you are willing to invest $30 a year to ensure you get enough of all the key vitamins, take a multivitamin.

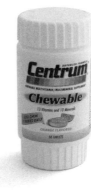

So that's:

- Fish

- Fiber

- Fruit and vegetables, and

- Folic acid.

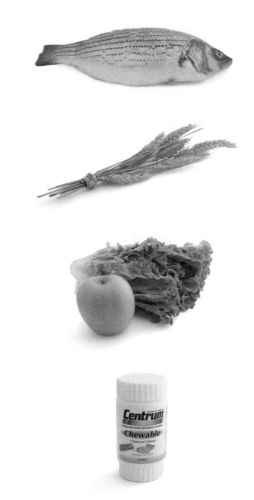

These are the four fine foods you
should favor.

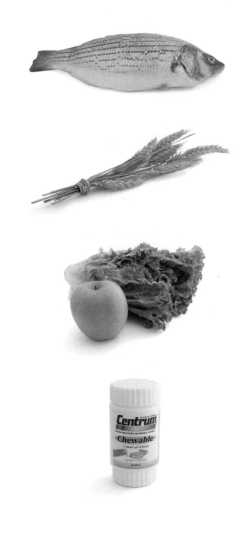

Compare that list with this list: the top 10 foods in terms of calories consumed in the US.

Together they account for one-third of all the energy consumed by Americans. If everyone substituted lower-calorie alternatives for just these 10, the obesity epidemic would disappear.

1	Bread	6.8%
2	Potato	5.1%
3	Milk	4.8%
4	Cola soft drink	3.4%
5	Beef	3.4%
6	Pizza	2.7%
7	Chicken	2.5%
8	Cheese	2.3%
9	Rice	2.0%
10	Cookies	2.0%

SOURCE: *1994-96, 1998 Continuing Survey of Food Intakes by Individuals*, USDA, www.barc.usda.gov/foodsurvey/home.htm

TWO

By now you should be able to make a good estimate of the calorie content of most foods.

These for instance: which has fewer calories, a glass of orange juice or an orange?

(Hint: a glass of orange juice has roughly the same number of calories as other drinks, thanks to the sugar.)

Orange juice = ?

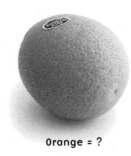

Orange = ?

The orange has fewer, 50.

You could guess that the orange juice is roughly 150 calories (140 for a 10-ounce glass, in fact).

So if you feel like a glass of orange juice, have an orange instead.

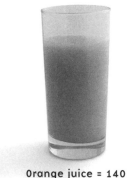

Orange juice = 140

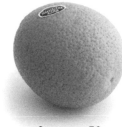

Orange = 50

And you can recognize a fitness opportunity when you see one.

This for instance: you are on a bus or subway, one stop from your destination, and you have some time to spare.

What might you do in this situation to get fitter?

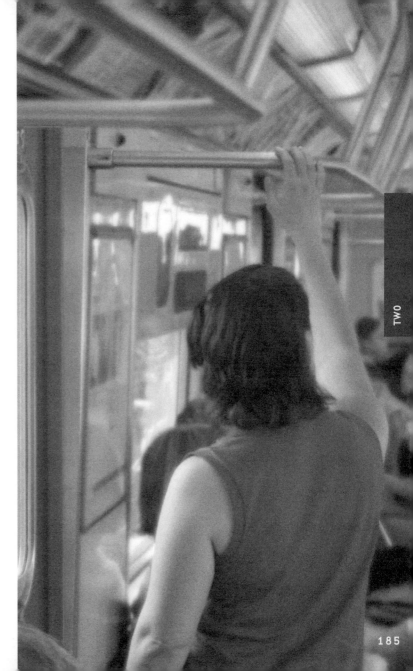

Get off a stop early and walk
(briskly) the rest of the way.

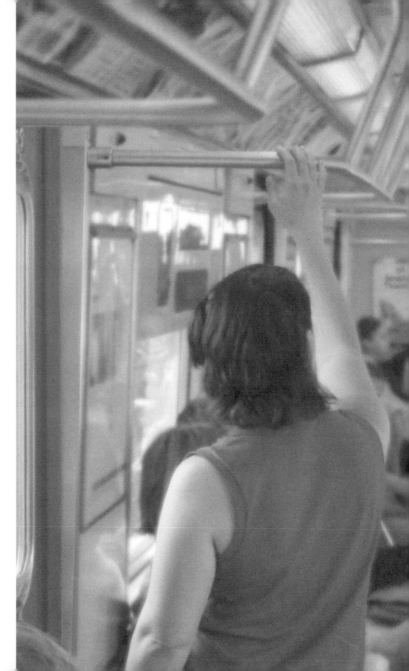

How many minutes of brisk walking do you need to do at least five days a week to reap most of the health benefits of exercise?

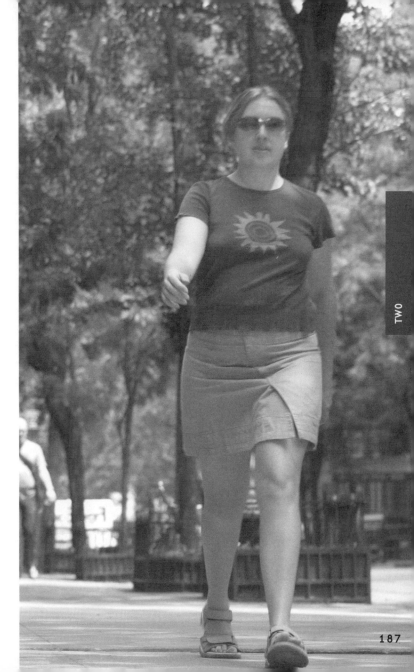

30 minutes.

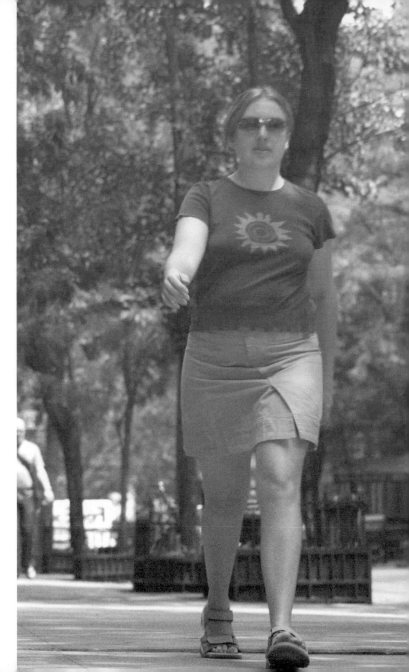

Finally, can you remember two
of the four fine foods you
should favor?

?

?

?

?

- Fish

- Fiber

- Fruit and vegetables, and

- Folic acid.

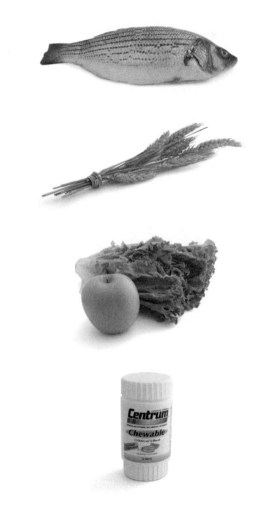

Good foods, bad foods, nutrition labels, and exercise —you can safely say you have a solid grounding in weight management.

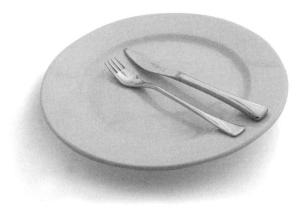

Certainly, you know enough to manage your own weight, avoid the bad stuff, and choose the good. Which is more than most people know.

Remember to practice your new skills within a week, or they will fade.

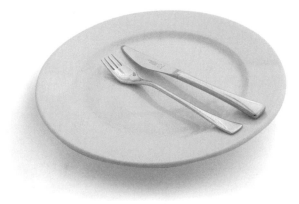

Pause point

Take a break after reading this page.

As before, you'll get most from this book if you stop here and return a few days later. If you can, get some practice by applying what you've learned to nutrition labels you come across and eating better foods.

The next section, the Epilogue, recaps everything you have learned so far. It doesn't introduce any new material; instead, it helps you hone your skills.

You know enough by now to find the Next Steps section interesting. It starts on page 229 and has pointers to a variety of resources you can use to build on the hooks you have installed in your head so far.

Epilogue

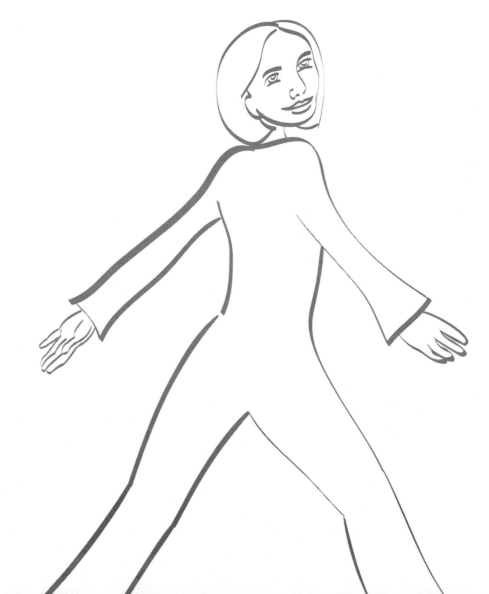

By now, you know far more than most people about weight management. You understand the simple principles that can be applied in a wide variety of situations.

Let's use this knowledge to analyze some of the most popular diets.

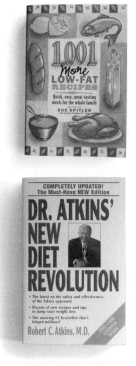

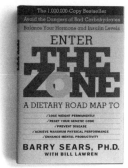

Followers of a 'low-fat diet' avoid all fatty food but don't worry too much about calories.

Is this a successful approach to losing weight, in your opinion?

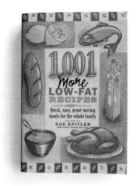

No. To lose weight you need to reduce calories, not fat. Fat in your diet does not translate directly into fat in your body.

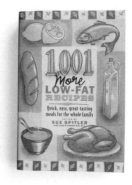

As we've seen, some low-fat foods have as many calories as their full-fat equivalents.

Also, cutting out all fat ignores the fact that some fat is good. It's cholesterol, saturated fat and trans fats that are bad for you.

The Atkins diet directs you to eat as much fat as you like but little or no carbohydrates (bread, potatoes, rice, etc).

Do you think this will work?

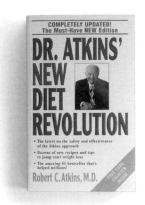

No, unless you cut calories too. The type of food you eat is far less important than how much energy it contains.

Some people do lose weight on an Atkins diet because it's difficult to maintain your calorie intake when you're not allowed bread, potatoes, or rice! But there is no evidence of a long-term change in metabolism so, when the diet is over, the weight lost may come right back. Meanwhile, all that bad fat could lead to heart disease.

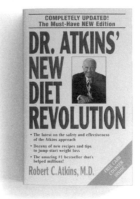

One more. To follow the Zone diet you have to consume the same number of calories from fat, protein, and carbohydrates each meal.

Do you think this will work?

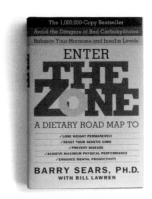

Again, unlikely—though people may eat less on the Zone diet just because it's so darned difficult to follow. But they often regain it when they come off the diet.

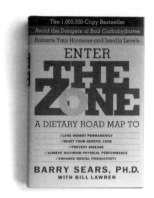

Which is why permanent substitutions work better. Instead of a yo-yo, on-again-off-again diet, you make small changes to your calorie intake that add up over time.

It's easy to see that these fad diets aren't working. If they were, Americans would be getting lighter, not heavier.

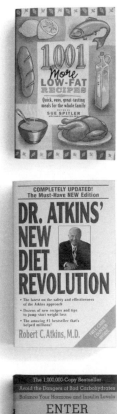

Here's a common problem: you're eating out and no Nutrition Facts are available.

LUNCH MENU

BURGERS, DOGS AND SANDWICHES

Hot Dog	$0.79	Grilled Cheese	$1.35
Hamburger	$1.70	Ham Sandwich (Deli)	$2.89
Cheeseburger	$1.95	Turkey Sandwich (Deli)	$2.89
Bacon Hamburger	$2.09	Club Sandwich	$3.69
Bacon Cheeseburger	$2.35	Chicken Salad (homemade)	$2.59
BBQ	$2.95	Tuna Salad (homemade)	$2.59
BLT	$1.89	Ribeye (4oz)	$2.89
		Grilled Chicken Breast	$2.59

SALADS

Small House Salad	$1.50	Large House Salad	$2.20
Small Chef Salad	$2.40	Large Chef Salad	$3.95
(Includes: Ham, Turkey & Cheese)			
Dressings: French, Thousand Island, Ranch & Blue Cheese			
Small Mixed Fruit Salad	$1.19	Large Mixed Fruit Salad	$1.49
Chicken Salad on Lettuce	$2.49		

SIDE ORDERS

French Fries	$0.99	Onion Rings	$1.09
Small Soup of the Day	$1.45	Large Soup of the Day	$1.95
Potato Salad	$0.99	Chicken Salad (lb.)	$4.89

SPECIALS

Hot Dog Special (Hot Dog, Fries, Med. Drink or Tea)	$2.69
2 Hot Dog Special (2 Hot Dogs, Fries, Med. Drink or Tea)	$3.39
Hamburger Special (Hamburger, Fries, Med. Drink or Tea)	$3.59
Cheeseburger Special (Cheeseburger, Fries, Med. Drink or Tea)	$3.79
1/2 Sandwich and Soup of the Day (Excludes Club Sandwiches)	$2.99
Ask about our "Special of the Day" (Mon-Fri)	

ASK ABOUT OUR HOMEMADE DESSERTS

BEVERAGES

Iced Tea	Med $0.89	Large	$1.09
Coffee			$0.75
Orange Juice			$0.99
Milk			$0.99
Coke, Diet Coke, Dr Pepper, Sprite	Med $0.89	Large	$1.09
(All to go soft drinks or tea 14oz $0.99)			

1 refill on Coffee, med. Tea or med. Soft Drink

Take a look at this menu, for instance.

Bearing in mind everything you now know, what would you choose for lunch?

LUNCH MENU

BURGERS, DOGS AND SANDWICHES

Hot Dog	$0.79	Grilled Cheese	$1.35
Hamburger	$1.70	Ham Sandwich (Deli)	$2.89
Cheeseburger	$1.95	Turkey Sandwich (Deli)	$2.89
Bacon Hamburger	$2.09	Club Sandwich	$3.69
Bacon Cheeseburger	$2.35	Chicken Salad (homemade)	$2.59
BBQ	$2.95	Tuna Salad (homemade)	$2.59
BLT	$1.89	Ribeye (4oz)	$2.89
		Grilled Chicken Breast	$2.59

SALADS

Small House Salad	$1.50	Large House Salad	$2.20
Small Chef Salad	$2.40	Large Chef Salad	$3.95
(Includes: Ham, Turkey & Cheese)			
Dressings: French, Thousand Island, Ranch & Blue Cheese			
Small Mixed Fruit Salad	$1.19	Large Mixed Fruit Salad	$1.49
Chicken Salad on Lettuce	$2.49		

SIDE ORDERS

French Fries	$0.99	Onion Rings	$1.09
Small Soup of the Day	$1.45	Large Soup of the Day	$1.95
Potato Salad	$0.99	Chicken Salad (lb.)	$4.89

SPECIALS

Hot Dog Special (Hot Dog, Fries, Med. Drink or Tea)	$2.69
2 Hot Dog Special (2 Hot Dogs, Fries, Med. Drink or Tea)	$3.39
Hamburger Special (Hamburger, Fries, Med. Drink or Tea)	$3.59
Cheeseburger Special (Cheeseburger, Fries, Med. Drink or Tea)	$3.79
1/2 Sandwich and Soup of the Day (Excludes Club Sandwiches)	$2.99
Ask about our "Special of the Day" (Mon-Fri)	

ASK ABOUT OUR HOMEMADE DESSERTS

BEVERAGES

Iced Tea	Med $0.89	Large $1.09
Coffee		$0.75
Orange Juice		$0.99
Milk		$0.99
Coke, Diet Coke, Dr Pepper, Sprite	Med $0.89	Large $1.09
(All to go soft drinks or tea 14oz $0.99)		

1 refill on Coffee, med. Tea or med. Soft Drink

Any salad is likely have lower calories than any sandwich. (Ask for a dressing with olive oil.)

If you think that may leave you vulnerable to a mid-afternoon snack attack, try a sandwich. Chicken, turkey, or tuna are best on this list.

And, of course, if the portions are large, you don't have to eat it all.

LUNCH MENU

BURGERS, DOGS AND SANDWICHES

Hot Dog	$0.79	Grilled Cheese	$1.35
Hamburger	$1.70	Ham Sandwich (Deli)	$2.89
Cheeseburger	$1.95	Turkey Sandwich (Deli)	$2.89
Bacon Hamburger	$2.09	Club Sandwich	$3.69
Bacon Cheeseburger	$2.35	Chicken Salad (homemade)	$2.59
BBQ	$2.95	Tuna Salad (homemade)	$2.59
BLT	$1.89	Ribeye (4oz)	$2.89
		Grilled Chicken Breast	$2.59

SALADS

Small House Salad	$1.50	Large House Salad	$2.20
Small Chef Salad	$2.40	Large Chef Salad	$3.95
(Includes: Ham, Turkey & Cheese)			

Dressings: French, Thousand Island, Ranch & Blue Cheese

Small Mixed Fruit Salad	$1.19	Large Mixed Fruit Salad	$1.49
Chicken Salad on Lettuce	$2.49		

SIDE ORDERS

French Fries	$0.99	Onion Rings	$1.09
Small Soup of the Day	$1.45	Large Soup of the Day	$1.95
Potato Salad	$0.99	Chicken Salad (lb.)	$4.89

SPECIALS

Hot Dog Special (Hot Dog, Fries, Med. Drink or Tea)	$2.69
2 Hot Dog Special (2 Hot Dogs, Fries, Med. Drink or Tea)	$3.39
Hamburger Special (Hamburger, Fries, Med. Drink or Tea)	$3.59
Cheeseburger Special (Cheeseburger, Fries, Med. Drink or Tea)	$3.79
1/2 Sandwich and Soup of the Day (Excludes Club Sandwiches)	$2.99

Ask about our "Special of the Day" (Mon-Fri)

ASK ABOUT OUR HOMEMADE DESSERTS

BEVERAGES

Iced Tea	Med $0.89		Large $1.09
Coffee			$0.75
Orange Juice			$0.99
Milk			$0.99
Coke, Diet Coke, Dr Pepper, Sprite	Med $0.89		Large $1.09

(All to go soft drinks or tea 14oz $0.99)

1 refill on Coffee, med. Tea or med. Soft Drink

Try this one.

Choose an appetizer and an entrée.

Tavolo d'Oro

APPETIZERS

HOMEMADE MINESTRONE (made from vegetable stock)	1.75	DINNER SALAD (mixed greens, carrots & peperoncini)	1.75
CREAM OF BROCCOLI SOUP (made from homemade chicken stock) (Soup to go)	1.75	LARGE ITALIAN SALAD	3.95
		SMALL ITALIAN SALAD	2.75
	2.00	(Italian Salads include mixed greens, carrots, red onion, cucumber, radish, provolone cheese & peperoncini) Served with our homemade Italian, Creamy Garlic, Balsamic (fat free) or 1000 Island Dressings. Extra salad ingredients or dressings .25 extra	
SPINACH SALAD (with mushroom & red onion in a tangy vinaigrette)	3.25		
CAESAR SALAD	3.95	GARLIC BREAD	1.50
CAESAR SALAD w/chicken	6.50		
GORGONZOLA SALAD (mixed greens, tomatoes & calamata olives)	3.25		

ENTREES

SPAGHETTI	6.50	SPAGHETTI DIABLO (Fresh Hot Peppers	7.95
MOSTACIOLI	6.50	sauteed in Garlic & Olive Oil with	11.50
ROTINI	6.50	Marinara Sauce)	
ANGEL HAIR	6.50	SPAGHETTI DIABLO w/SHRIMP	8.50
HOMEMADE SPINACH ROTINI	6.75	SPAGHETTI MARINARA PRIMAVERA	7.50
RAVIOLI (filled w/Spinach & 4 cheeses)	8.50	(w/Broccoli, Carrots &	
BAKED SPAGHETTI with	7.50	Red Bell Peppers)	
MOZZARELLA CHEESE		SPAGHETTI PESTO	11.50
The above are served with your choice of		FETTUCINE ALFREDO	8.25
Meat, Marinara or Butter & Garlic Sauce.		FETTUCINE ALFREDO w/SHRIMP	9.50
SPAGHETTI AGLIO E OLIO	7.50	FETTUCINE ALFREDO w/DICED	8.25
(Garlic & Olive Oil)		CHICKEN BREAST	
SPAGHETTI CARBONARA (Bacon &	8.50	FETTUCINE ALFREDO PRIMAVERA	8.25
Onion in a Cream & Egg Sauce)		(Broccoli, Carrots & Red Bell Peppers)	
SPAGHETTI GORGONZOLA (a creamy	8.50	Any sauce w/Mushrooms	.75 extra
blue cheese sauce)		Meatball (1/4 lb. uncooked)	
SPAGHETTI WHITE CLAM SAUCE	8.25	if ordered with entree	1.50 extra
(creamy style)		ordered separately	2.25 extra
SPAGHETTI RED CLAM SAUCE	8.25	Italian Sausage	
SPAGHETTI CALAMARI (sliced squid	9.50	(if ordered with entree)	1.95 extra
sauteed in Garlic & Olive Oil with		ordered separately	3.50 extra
Marinara Sauce)			

Soup is a good choice, preferably avoiding cream. Or salad, avoiding cheese.

All the pasta dishes could be a similar number of calories; how many you consume will depend more on the size of the serving and how much of it you eat.

Tavolo d'Oro

APPETIZERS

HOMEMADE MINESTRONE (made from vegetable stock)	1.75	DINNER SALAD (mixed greens, carrots & peperoncini)	1.75
CREAM OF BROCCOLI SOUP (made from homemade chicken stock)	1.75	LARGE ITALIAN SALAD	3.95
(Soup to go)	2.00	SMALL ITALIAN SALAD	2.75
SPINACH SALAD (with mushroom & red onion in a tangy vinaigrette)	3.25	(Italian Salads include mixed greens, carrots, red onion, cucumber, radish, provolone cheese & peperoncini) Served with our homemade Italian, Creamy Garlic, Balsamic (fat free) or 1000 Island Dressings. Extra salad ingredients or dressings .25 extra	
CAESAR SALAD	3.95		
CAESAR SALAD w/chicken	6.50	GARLIC BREAD	1.50
GORGONZOLA SALAD (mixed greens, tomatoes & calamata olives)	3.25		

ENTREES

SPAGHETTI	6.50	SPAGHETTI DIABLO (Fresh Hot Peppers	7.95
MOSTACIOLI	6.50	sauteed in Garlic & Olive Oil with	11.50
ROTINI	6.50	Marinara Sauce)	
ANGEL HAIR	6.50	SPAGHETTI DIABLO w/SHRIMP	8.50
HOMEMADE SPINACH ROTINI	6.75	SPAGHETTI MARINARA PRIMAVERA	7.50
RAVIOLI (filled w/Spinach & 4 cheeses)	8.50	(w/Broccoli, Carrots &	
BAKED SPAGHETTI with	7.50	Red Bell Peppers)	
MOZZARELLA CHEESE		SPAGHETTI PESTO	11.50
The above are served with your choice of		FETTUCINE ALFREDO	8.25
Meat, Marinara or Butter & Garlic Sauce.		FETTUCINE ALFREDO w/SHRIMP	9.50
SPAGHETTI AGLIO E OLIO	7.50	FETTUCINE ALFREDO w/DICED	8.25
(Garlic & Olive Oil)		CHICKEN BREAST	
SPAGHETTI CARBONARA (Bacon &	8.50	FETTUCINE ALFREDO PRIMAVERA	8.25
Onion in a Cream & Egg Sauce)		(Broccoli, Carrots & Red Bell Peppers)	
SPAGHETTI GORGONZOLA (a creamy	8.50	Any sauce w/Mushrooms	.75 extra
blue cheese sauce)		Meatball (1/4 lb. uncooked)	
SPAGHETTI WHITE CLAM SAUCE	8.25	if ordered with entree	1.50 extra
(creamy style)		ordered separately	2.25 extra
SPAGHETTI RED CLAM SAUCE	8.25	Italian Sausage	
SPAGHETTI CALAMARI (sliced squid	9.50	(if ordered with entree)	1.95 extra
sauteed in Garlic & Olive Oil with		ordered separately	3.50 extra
Marinara Sauce)			

Okay, the grand finale.

How many calories in this
candy bar?

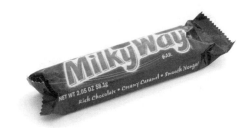

250.

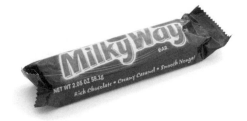

A substitution: instead of a soda,
an orange. How many calories
do you save?

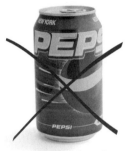

12-oz soda = ?

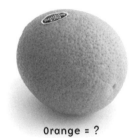

Orange = ?

100.

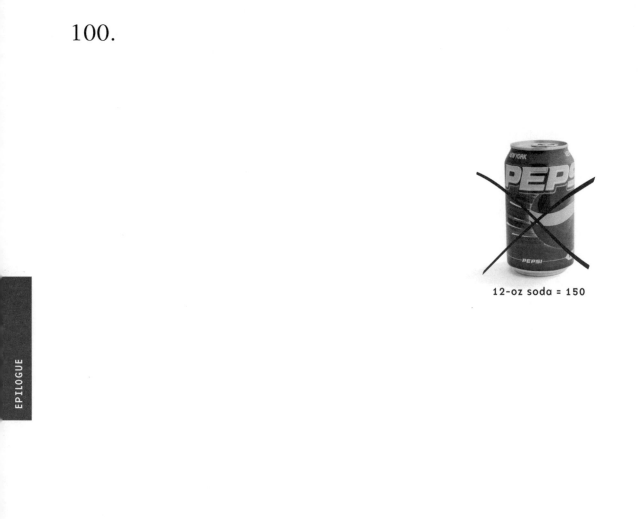

12-oz soda = 150

Orange = 50

Which four of these twelve
foods should you favor?

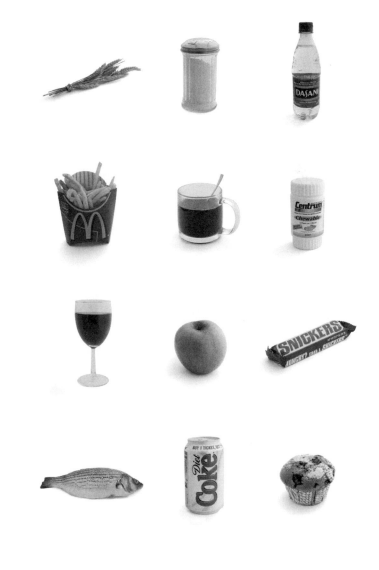

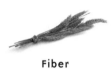

Fiber

Folic acid

Fruit (and
vegetables)

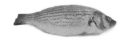

Fish

Which one of these twelve is
most likely to contain trans fat?

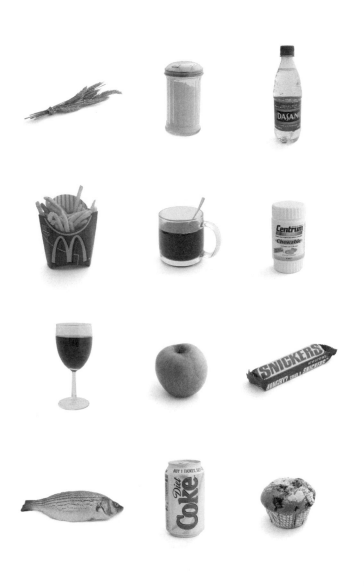

The fries.

Did you know that, in Scotland, deep fried candy is a popular snack? So if you are Scottish, you could also have chosen the Snickers.

Deep fried food

What five areas are of most interest on a Nutrition Facts label?

Nutrition Facts

Serving Size 1 oz (28g/About 20 chips)
Servings Per Container About 6

Amount Per Serving

Calories 150	Calories from Fat 90

	% Daily Value*
Total Fat 10g	**15**%
Saturated Fat 3g	**15**%
Cholesterol 0mg	**0**%
Sodium 180mg	**8**%
Total Carbohydrate 15g	**5**%
Dietary Fiber 1g	**4**%
Sugars 0g	
Protein 2g	

Vitamin A 0%	•	Vitamin C 10%
Calcuim 0%	•	Iron 0%

* Percent Daily Values are based on a 2,000 calorie diet.
  Your daily values may be higher or lower depending
  on your calorie needs:

	Calories:	2,000	2,500
Total Fat	Less than	65g	80g
Sat Fat	Less than	20g	25g
Cholesterol	Less than	300mg	300mg
Sodium	Less than	2,400mg	2,400mg
Total Carbohydrate		300g	375g
Dietary Fiber		25g	30g

Calories per gram: Fat 9 • Carbohydrate 4 • Protein 4

Serving size, calories, sat fat, cholesterol, and fiber.

(Whenever these give conflicting signals—such as a food with low sat fat but high calories—choose the food with the *lowest calories*.)

Nutrition Facts

Serving Size 1 oz (28g/About 20 chips)
Servings Per Container About 6

Amount Per Serving

Calories 150   Calories from Fat 90

% Daily Value*

Total Fat 10g	**15%**
Saturated Fat 3g	**15%**
Cholesterol 0mg	**0%**
Sodium 180mg	**8%**
Total Carbohydrate 15g	**5%**
Dietary Fiber 1g	**4%**
Sugars 0g	
Protein 2g	

Vitamin A 0%	•	Vitamin C 10%
Calcuim 0%	•	Iron 0%

* Percent Daily Values are based on a 2,000 calorie diet.
Your daily values may be higher or lower depending
on your calorie needs:

	Calories:	2,000	2,500
Total Fat	Less than	65g	80g
Sat Fat	Less than	20g	25g
Cholesterol	Less than	300mg	300mg
Sodium	Less than	2,400mg	2,400mg
Total Carbohydrate		300g	375g
Dietary Fiber		25g	30g

Calories per gram: Fat 9 • Carbohydrate 4 • Protein 4

Name any one of the three
tactics for dealing with hunger
and satiety.

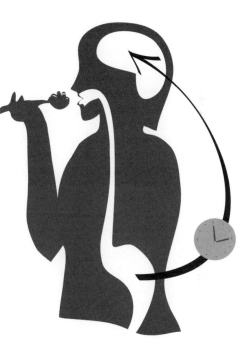

The three tactics are:

1. Stop eating *before* you are full.

2. Don't eat if you're not hungry.

3. Avoid leaving tempting food around.

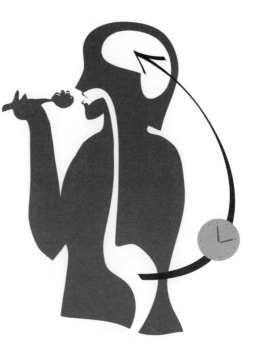

While out and about you
come across an escalator.
What should you do?

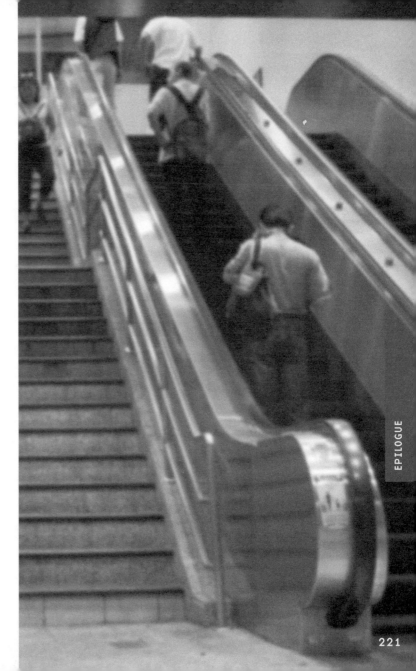

Take the stairs.

(Same with moving walkways
—see them as a signal to walk
briskly alongside.)

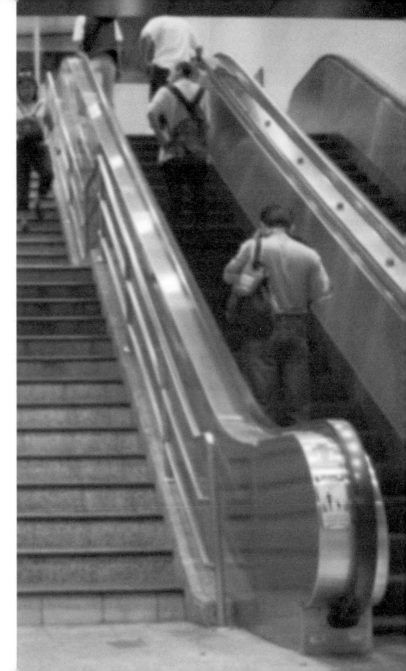

If you have read each page up to this one, you know how to gradually adjust your weight to where you want it. And how to keep it there while eating all the good stuff you want to eat (just not so much of it).

Spread of Obesity (Center for Disease Control). Darker shading means more obesity.

2001

The obesity explosion is very recent; any explanation for it must hinge on factors that are recent too.

For instance, the fact that calories have never been cheaper than they are in the US today. Nor has daily life ever been less physically demanding for most people.

Five years earlier, 1996.

So we are the first generations
to need the new skills of
weight management.

There is no mystery to it;
no miracle needed. The only
two ways to lose weight are
to eat fewer calories or
to burn more.

Of course, some people
will find this easier
than others.

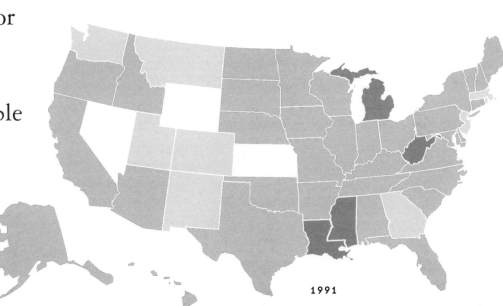

1991

But if you believe that the real you is underneath, healthier and happier, you owe it to that person to release them.

They will thank you.

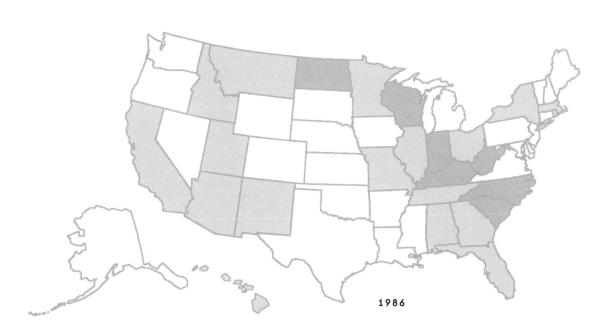

1986

Next Steps

Now that you know the basics of weight management, there is much more you can explore. We've included enough here to keep you busy and there is more, including references, at www.stikky.com/weightman, which is updated frequently.

Calorie counters

By now you have a good handle on the number of calories in common foods—but there will be some things you eat regularly that we didn't have space to cover.

- There are two copies (so you can pull one out) of a calorie table starting after page 234. It includes the 200 most commonly eaten foods in the US.

- Several websites, such as www.nutri-facts.com, have nutrition facts for most foods, and the Nutrient Data Laboratory maintains a database of food composition (not just calories, everything, even ash) at www.nal.usda.gov/fnic/foodcomp, though it is weak on brand name foods. (Note that some sources quote the energy content of foods in both *kcal*, which is the same thing as *calories*, and *kj*, which is not, so ignore it.)

- Allan Borushek's book *Doctor's Pocket Calories, Fat & Carbohydrate Counter* is small enough to carry around and includes both generic foods (pizza) and brand names (Domino's, Pizza Hut).

Measuring your progress

On any long-term venture, feedback is essential to maintain your motivation. There is nothing quite so heartening as making a change to your diet and finding, only a week or so later, that it has started to work. For that you need an accurate **scale**.

- To find out if a scale is accurate, weigh yourself three times in a row. If the highest and lowest weights differ by more than a few ounces, get a new scale.

- Your weight varies during the day, so always weigh yourself at the same time of day, preferably first thing in the morning, on the same scale, wearing as little as possible.

- Take a picture of yourself—the change to how you look is gradual, so friends can't be relied upon to notice.

- Keep monitoring your weight even after reaching your target, especially if you change job or house or something else that could alter your activity and eating patterns. It's a lot easier to correct a gain of two pounds than a gain of ten.

Some people like to measure their body fat as well as their weight, to ensure they are losing fat not muscle. Previously this involved skin fold calipers but these are difficult to use accurately. Now it's a cinch if you buy a scale with a **body fat monitor** built in, a feature popularized by Tanita (www.tanita.com). Their accuracy is not perfect but good enough to track fat reduction as you lose weight. Body fat above 25% for women and 20% for men has been linked to health problems.

A cheaper solution is a **tape measure**—there is evidence that waist circumference, in particular, is a very good indicator of health risk. Danger has been shown to exist above 33 inches for women and 35 inches for men. Measure your waist while you are standing: halfway between the bottom of your sternum (your breastbone, to which your ribs are attached) and your navel (your belly button). The tape should be snug but not pinching.

Measuring your burn rate

If you could burn more energy, you wouldn't need to cut as much from your diet. Many Americans burn so little energy that increasing it may not be difficult, especially if they could see when they're burning more. Two tools that help you do so are pedometers and heart rate monitors.

A **pedometer** is a low-cost device you wear all day, clipped onto your belt or pocket, that counts your steps. The equivalent of 30 minutes brisk walking (the daily recommended minimum) is 10,000 steps. So, if it's afternoon and your pedometer shows only 5,000 steps, you might plan a walk after dinner. Alternatively, measure your typical daily step count and try to beat it each day.

If you plan more vigorous activity such as a bike ride, jog, swim, aerobics, etc, a **heart rate monitor** is an excellent investment. The market leader is Polar (www.polarusa.com) but there are several other brands and all have similar features.

The benefit of a heart rate monitor is that it tells you how hard you are working—the higher your heart rate, the more calories you burn. To correct three exercise myths:

- There is no special 'fat burn' heart rate zone.

- Vigorous exercise carries a very small increased risk of sudden death (an extra one death per 1.5 million exercise sessions according to a study in 2000); the long-term benefits of exercise outweigh this risk.

- You cannot 'spot reduce' fat from a particular area of your body—so doing sit-ups burns fat from all over—but you can spot increase muscles through resistance training (for instance, using weights).

Diet-tracking sites and software

When your weight is stable, what you consume and what you burn must be the same. So, if you were able to track how many calories you consumed when your weight was stable for, say, two weeks, you would know how many calories you typically burn. Then you could figure out exactly what change to make to your diet to achieve your target weight. In the last few years, this has become possible for those with a computer and a little discipline.

- PC-based packages include *DietPower* (www.dietpower.com), *Performance Diet Pro* (www.health-runr.com), and *Diet & Exercise Assistant* (www.keyoe.com).

- Hand-held (PDA) applications have the advantage that you can have them with you whenever you are eating. They include *Diet Diary* (www.calorieking.com) and *Diet & Exercise Assistant* (www.keyoe.com) which synchronizes with the PC application of the same name.

- Web-based diet programs currently take a less helpful approach: instead of calculating your burn rate they guess it and focus instead on custom meal plans (usually of the grapefruit and broccoli variety, or so it seems).

Tests you or your doctor can do

You may have specific medical conditions that your diet should take into account. A first step, even if you don't suspect a particular medical problem, is to take the screening tests. Since the conditions are partly genetic, taking a test is especially important if you have a blood relative with one of them. Remember that general practitioners cover a vast range of diseases and may not be masters of any of them, so it's worth reading the full directions on interpreting results yourself.

- **Blood pressure tests** can be accurately performed at home with relatively inexpensive equipment. To interpret the results visit www.nhlbi.nih.gov/hbp.

- A **cholesterol test** reports the total cholesterol level in your blood and breaks it down into HDL (which is good, think Highly Desirable), LDL (bad, think Less Desirable), and triglycerides. If the test your doctor offers does not report all four numbers, request one that does (or buy a home test that does). Then go to www.nhlbi.nih.gov/guidelines/cholesterol which includes the comprehensive report of the National Cholesterol Education Program's Adult Treatment Panel.

- The main **blood sugar tests** are the Fasting Glucose Test, which measures the glucose level in your blood after at least eight hours of not eating, and the Oral Glucose Tolerance Test, which measures the level two hours after consuming a precise amount of sugar, and is only needed if the Fasting test is outside the normal range. (According to the American Diabetes Association, a urine test is inadequate for diagnosing diabetes and 'pre-diabetes'; request a blood test.) To interpret the results go to www.diabetes.org or call 1-800-DIABETES.

Specific foods

There is a danger, when focusing on the miracle or mischief of an individual nutrient, in getting too hung up on dietary fine-tuning. For the average American, the likely health benefit of consuming more calcium, say, is small and still a subject of dispute compared to the known benefits of being at or below target weight or quitting smoking.

Several thousand research papers are published every year. Since not all of them make the news, you can easily wind up with only part of the story for any single food. This section attempts to bring you up to date on foods not covered in the main text.

To find out which foods contain a particular nutrient, go to www.nal.usda.gov/fnic/foodcomp, 'Reports by Single Nutrients'.

Alcohol, any alcohol, reduces the risk of heart disease. But too much alcohol increases the risk of liver disease, some cancers, high blood pressure, stroke, and more. The optimum balance between these varies. On average it is no more than two drinks a day for men, especially older men with a high risk of heart disease, and one-to-two drinks for women unless they are pregnant or have a blood relative with breast cancer. A 'drink' means one unit: roughly half a glass of beer, half a glass of wine, or a shot of spirit.

Evidence is now strong that oxidation plays a role in heart disease, cancer, cataracts, and possibly Alzheimer's and other diseases, so **antioxidants** are important. Fruits and vegetables are cleverly designed packages of antioxidants, together with other good stuff. Exactly which antioxidant is responsible for which benefit is still poorly understood and miracle claims (such as those made for beta-carotene, presumably in an effort to save people from having to eat plants) have not stood up to full-blown studies. Until they do, plants rule.

There is a terrible confusion over **artificial sweeteners**, which is unfortunate since they offer an easy way to save 150 calories per can of soda. The confusion exists because an early sweetener, saccharin ("SACK-a-rin"), was found to cause cancer in lab rats. No such link has been found in humans, though it has not been ruled out for people who use six or more servings of saccharin a day. It is still used in Sweet 'n Low and in some fountain sodas. Aspartame ("AS-per-tame"), the sweetener in diet sodas, NutraSweet, and Equal, is one of the most thoroughly tested food additives in history and has proven safe for everyone except people with phenylketonuria (1 in 16,000). It is 180 times sweeter than sugar, so the amount in a can of soda is tiny.

Aspirin has been demonstrated to reduce the risk of heart disease. The American Heart Association recommends a low dose of aspirin daily for those with a 10% or greater risk of heart disease in the next 10 years. For anyone else, this benefit may be outweighed by the possibility of gastrointestinal bleeding.

Calcium helps prevent osteoporosis, reducing the risk of bone fracture, but the connection is not a straightforward one. Studies of people who consume the recommended amount of calcium (as the average American does) but who remain completely immobile, show rapid bone loss—so calcium alone is not enough. And people in countries that consume far less calcium per head than the US do not have more hip fractures. At the same time, some studies suggest that too much calcium may have a harmful effect with possible links to prostate and ovarian cancer. And, if your main source of calcium is dairy products,

you are taking in harmful saturated fat at the same time. So what else can you do to avoid osteoporosis?

- Training with weights strengthens bones and any exercise improves balance so you're less likely to fall and break something.

- Hormone replacement therapy is an option, mainly for women

- Vitamin D helps you absorb calcium and people who live. further north than San Francisco-Denver-Philadelphia may get too little direct sunlight to prompt the body to make its own; they may benefit from a vitamin D supplement.

- If you think you don't get enough calcium (perhaps because you have sensibly cut down on dairy products), take a supplement or eat foods such as calcium-set tofu, calcium-fortified juice, or broccoli.

Claims that calcium is a 'superstar nutrient', reducing hypertension and even reversing colon cancer, are unproven. Some studies have found intriguing results, but other studies were unable to reproduce them. Even so, exaggerated claims for coral calcium led to thousands of people over-paying for it.

Cholesterol in your diet leads to higher LDL (Less Desirable) cholesterol levels in your blood, increasing your risk of heart disease. The effect varies widely for different people; some can get away with it. Major sources of cholesterol include eggs, meat, dairy products, and some fish. Plants contain no cholesterol.

Coffee increases your blood pressure, but the effect is short-lived and no link has been found between drinking coffee and heart disease. Filter coffee and instant coffee are considered safe and may even benefit health. Espresso and French press coffee may increase cholesterol a little.

Eggs are a major source of cholesterol but, oddly, research has not linked egg consumption to heart disease, perhaps because they contain a lot of beneficial nutrients too. So eggs are a sort of in-between food—fruit is better for you, but cheese is worse.

As featured in the main text, **folic acid** is the vitamin people lack for which the best evidence of health benefits exists. Pregnant women who get too little folic acid increase the risk of neural-tube defects in their child. Folic acid is also linked to decreased risk of heart disease, colon cancer, and breast cancer. Good sources include fortified breakfast cereals, lentils, spinach, and pasta.

Foods containing carbohydrate with a high **glycemic index** (GI) turn into sugar faster once eaten, which can cause diabetes. Most refined foods, like white bread or corn flakes, have a high GI (http://diabetes.about.com/library/mendosagi/ngilists.htm lists the GI of just about everything). Fiber reduces a food's GI. Researchers figured out, as recently as the 1980s, that the spike in blood sugar you get after eating high GI carbohydrate triggers a spike in insulin which, in turn, reduces your blood sugar so sharply that you feel hungry again within a couple of hours. If you then eat another high GI snack, the cycle starts again. This glucose-insulin roller-coaster can exacerbate a condition called the metabolic syndrome (or 'syndrome X'), a combination of overweight, insulin-resistance, and risk of heart disease. So a diet high in the wrong sort of carbohydrate (including the diet recommended in the USDA Food Pyramid) could be as dangerous as one high in the wrong sort of fat. The definitive book on this topic is Gerry Reaven's *Syndrome X*.

There is not enough evidence yet to justify increasing intake of **minerals** other than iron for infants and pre-menopausal women. Potassium (in bananas, baked beans, tomatoes, etc) can lower blood pressure, though too much is harmful. Cutting back on sodium (eg, salt) can also lower blood pressure for some. Zinc, contrary to some reports, does not cure the common cold.

N-3 fatty acid (also known as omega-3 fatty acid) is a type of unsaturated fat found mostly in fatty fish such as salmon, sardine, trout, swordfish, herring, mackerel, halibut, and tuna (in that order). It is also available in fish oil pills. It is an 'essential' fat (meaning your body can't make it) and has recently been found to cut sudden cardiac death by half in people who have suffered a previous heart attack. In one study, one gram of n-3 a day produced a significant effect within four months.

A link between **nuts** and reduced risk of heart disease has recently been established. But there's a problem: nuts are packed with calories (1.5 ounces of peanuts or peanut butter has the same number of calories as a Snickers) and are often laced with salt. Substitute them for chips or candy or for meat in your main meal.

Soy products make for excellent substitutions because soy is low in calories and saturated fat. Ounce for ounce, tofu has less than half the calories and a quarter of the sat fat of chicken. There may be other benefits, but you have to eat a lot of soy; participants in a study linking soy to lower LDL cholesterol ate the equivalent of 1.5 pounds of tofu a day. Hints of possible downsides from soy, such as memory loss, are unproven.

Vitamins are nutrients you need but your body can't make—you have to get them from food. Vitamin deficiency has been known for a long time to cause scurvy and rickets (not common in the US today). More recently, some cancers and heart disease have been linked to vitamin deficiency. The evidence is still unfolding but there is wide agreement that most people would benefit from more: folic acid, B$_6$, B$_{12}$, D, and, for those at risk of coronary disease, E. Most multivitamins contain the recommended daily amount of all these. A good piece on multivitamins is at www.cspinet.org/nah/01_03/spin.pdf. (Oh, and extra vitamin C, contrary to reports, neither prevents nor cures colds.)

Since **water** contains zero calories, it's a great substitution for any other drink. But claims that you need to drink eight 8oz glasses a day are a nutrition myth.

Books, websites, newsletters

There are plenty of outstandingly poor books on diet and nutrition. But there are also a few good ones: *Eat, Drink, and Be Healthy* by Walter Willett, *The Volumetrics Weight-Control Plan* by Barbara Rolls and Robert Barnett, *Syndrome X* by Gerry Reaven, and *The Burn Rate Diet* by Stephen Van Scholyck.

Fascinating reads on the search for obesity causes and cures are Robert Pool's *Fat: Fighting the Obesity Epidemic* and Ellen Ruppel Shell's *The Hungry Gene*. The conclusions are worth relating:

- Drug and gene therapies for obesity in the general population are several years away and likely to be unattractive (requiring daily injections, for instance).

- Obesity is most often due to faulty internal regulation of eating, driven partly by genes and partly by how you ate when you were young (the same things that determine your height).

- The cure is most likely part environmental (food manufacturers need to provide better options) and part helping people develop the cognitive skills to eat less and lounge less.

The internet is a hazardous place to seek nutrition information —be skeptical of any article that doesn't quote references.

- MEDLINEplus (www.medlineplus.gov) allows you to search the huge National Library of Medicine, which includes research on the health effects of just about any food.

- You can also search the medical papers themselves (including references given in our online Insider pages) at Medline, www.ncbi.nlm.nih.gov/entrez/query.fcgi. Abstracts, with conclusions, are free. The full papers can get technical, but this is the work that everything else (other than fiction) is based on.

- WebMD (www.webmd.com), though mainly a health site, is very thorough and up to date on diet and nutrition.

- The US government sadly has a tainted reputation for nutrition information, since the US Department of Agriculture. (www.usda.gov/cnpp) is responsible for food production as well as consumption, apparently in that order. (A fascinating exposé on the flawed process for designing the famous Food Pyramid is in Marion Nestle's book *Food Politics*.) The numerous government nutrition sites are cataloged at www.nutrition.gov.

- The Food and Drug Administration publishes a consumer magazine (free at www.fda.gov/fdac) which is dry but solid.

Two subscription newsletters worth a look are *Nutrition Action*, known for its stridency, published by The Center for Science in the Public Interest (http://cspinet.org/nah) and *Tufts University Health & Nutrition Newsletter* (http://healthletter.tufts.edu).

America's 200 Most Commonly Eaten Foods

Rank		Grams	Calories	Sat Fat	Cholesterol	Fiber	Folate	Vitamin B6	Vitamin B12	Vitamin E	Calcium	Iron	Potassium	Sodium
		g	kcal	g	mg	g	mg	mg	mcg	ATE	mg	mg	mg	mg
17	**Apple,** raw, 1 medium large (2-3/4", 4.9 oz)	138.0	81.4	0.1	0.0	3.73	3.9	0.07	0.00	0.4	9.7	0.25	158.7	0.0
169	**Bacon,** 1 medium slice (0.3 oz cooked)	8.0	46.1	1.4	6.8	0.00	0.4	0.02	0.14	0.0	1.0	0.13	38.9	127.7
123	**Bagel,** 1 medium (2-3/4" to 3-1/4", 2 oz)	57.0	156.8	0.1	0.0	1.31	50.2	0.03	0.00	0.0	42.2	2.03	57.6	304.4
94	**Bagel,** toasted, 1 medium (2-3/4" to 3-1/4", 1.9 oz)	53.0	156.4	0.1	0.0	1.33	39.8	0.03	0.00	0.0	42.4	2.02	57.8	304.2
12	**Banana,** 1 medium (7" to 7-7/8" long, 4.2 oz)	118.0	108.6	0.2	0.0	2.83	22.5	0.68	0.00	0.3	7.1	0.37	467.3	1.2
91	**Barbecue sauce,** 1 packet (0.3 fl oz)	9.3	7.0	0.0	0.0	0.11	0.4	0.01	0.00	0.1	1.8	0.08	16.2	75.8
117	**Beans,** green, 10 beans (2.2 oz)	62.0	12.4	0.0	0.0	1.18	18.7	0.02	0.00	0.1	16.1	0.56	67.6	162.4
104	**Beef,** ground, lean, 1 medium patty (4 oz, raw, 3.1 oz cooked)	88.0	237.4	6.3	75.9	0.00	7.9	0.23	2.05	0.2	9.8	1.84	262.7	351.3
57	**Beef,** ground, regular, 1 medium patty (4 oz, raw, 3 oz cooked)	85.0	243.6	6.9	75.9	0.00	7.6	0.23	2.47	0.2	9.4	2.06	246.2	344.4
95	**Beef,** patty, 1 medium patty (4 oz, raw, 3 oz cooked)	85.0	232.1	6.3	73.8	0.00	7.6	0.22	2.15	0.2	8.7	1.94	253.0	340.1
124	**Beef,** roasted, lean only, 1 medium slice (4-1/2" x 2-1/2" x 1/4", 1.5 oz)	42.0	82.9	1.4	32.3	0.00	3.4	0.14	1.07	0.1	2.6	1.08	158.0	96.1
82	**Beef steak,** broiled or baked, lean only, 1 medium steak (5.5 oz cooked)	156.0	307.5	4.7	125.1	0.00	14.4	0.71	3.93	0.2	13.8	4.27	636.4	605.2
122	**Biscuit,** baking powder or buttermilk type, 1 regular biscuit (0.7 oz)	19.0	65.7	0.7	0.0	0.30	8.2	0.01	0.00	0.3	3.8	0.49	29.8	228.4
168	**Biscuit,** McDonald's, 1 biscuit (2.5 oz)	72.0	262.1	1.8	0.7	0.94	42.5	0.03	0.10	2.1	35.3	2.38	161.3	757.4
136	**Bologna,** 1 medium slice (4-1/2" dia x 1/8" thick, 1 oz)	28.4	89.6	3.0	15.6	0.00	1.4	0.05	0.38	0.1	3.4	0.43	51.0	288.9
186	**Bread,** French or Vienna, 1 medium slice (4-3/4" x 4" x 1/2", 0.9 oz)	25.0	68.5	0.2	0.0	0.75	23.8	0.01	0.00	0.1	18.8	0.63	28.3	152.3
161	**Bread,** Italian, Grecian, Armenian, 1 medium slice (0.7 oz)	20.0	54.2	0.2	0.0	0.54	19.0	0.01	0.00	0.1	15.6	0.59	22.0	116.8
147	**Bread,** rye, 1 regular slice (0.9 oz)	26.0	67.3	0.2	0.0	1.51	22.4	0.02	0.00	0.1	19.0	0.74	43.2	171.6
8	**Bread,** white, 1 regular slice (0.9 oz)	26.0	69.4	0.1	0.3	0.60	24.7	0.02	0.01	0.1	28.1	0.79	30.9	139.9
23	**Bread,** white, toasted, 1 regular slice (0.8 oz)	23.0	67.4	0.1	0.2	0.58	15.8	0.01	0.00	0.1	27.4	0.77	30.1	136.2
38	**Bread,** whole wheat, 100%, 1 regular slice (1 oz)	28.0	68.9	0.3	0.0	1.93	14.0	0.05	0.00	0.3	20.2	0.92	70.6	147.6
77	**Bread,** whole wheat, 100%, toasted, 1 regular slice (0.9 oz)	25.0	69.3	0.3	0.0	1.85	9.8	0.05	0.00	0.2	20.3	0.93	70.8	148.0
135	**Bread,** whole wheat, other than 100%, 1 regular slice (0.9 oz)	26.0	67.6	0.2	0.0	1.12	20.0	0.03	0.00	0.1	27.3	0.86	52.3	137.8
200	**Bread,** whole wheat, other than 100%, toasted, 1 regular slice (0.9 oz)	24.0	67.7	0.2	0.0	1.27	15.6	0.02	0.00	0.1	27.4	0.86	52.3	138.2
112	**Bread, roll,** hoagie, submarine, 1 medium (8" long, 3.3 oz)	94.0	268.8	1.1	0.0	2.54	119.4	0.04	0.06	1.5	130.7	2.98	132.5	526.4
197	**Bread, roll,** sweet, cinnamon bun, frosted, 1 medium (2" - 2-1/2", 1.9 oz)	55.0	208.5	1.6	29.1	1.06	22.9	0.05	0.06	1.4	33.1	0.71	50.9	193.8
9	**Bread, roll,** white, soft, 1 large hamburger, frankfurter, onion roll (1.5 oz)	43.0	123.0	0.5	0.0	1.16	54.6	0.02	0.03	0.7	59.8	1.36	60.6	240.8
174	**Broccoli,** cooked, from fresh, 1 cup flowerets (3.4 oz)	97.0	27.0	0.1	0.0	2.80	48.2	0.14	0.00	1.6	44.5	0.81	281.6	255.0
29	**Butter,** stick, salted, 1 tablespoon (0.5 oz)	14.2	101.8	7.2	31.1	0.00	0.4	0.00	0.02	0.2	3.4	0.02	3.7	117.3
96	**Butter,** stick, unsalted, 1 tablespoon (0.5 oz)	14.2	101.8	7.2	31.1	0.00	0.4	0.00	0.02	0.2	3.3	0.02	3.7	1.6
66	**Cantaloupe** (muskmelon), 1 wedge (1/8 of medium melon, 2.4 oz)	69.0	24.2	0.0	0.0	0.55	11.7	0.08	0.00	0.1	7.6	0.14	213.2	6.2
26	**Carrot,** raw, 1 small (5-1/2" long, 1.75 oz)	50.0	21.5	0.0	0.0	1.50	7.0	0.07	0.00	0.1	13.5	0.25	161.5	17.5
88	**Celery,** 1 medium stalk (7-1/2" - 8" long) (1.4 oz)	40.0	6.4	0.0	0.0	0.68	11.2	0.03	0.00	0.1	16.0	0.16	114.8	34.8
90	**Cheerios,** 1 cup (1.1 oz)	30.0	109.5	0.4	0.0	2.64	99.9	0.50	0.00	0.2	55.2	8.10	88.5	284.1
24	**Cheese,** Cheddar or American type, processed, 1 slice (1 oz)	28.4	95.0	4.6	19.4	0.00	2.1	0.04	0.30	0.2	164.5	0.22	74.4	346.9
54	**Cheese,** Cheddar or American type, 1 slice (0.85 oz)	24.0	85.7	4.3	19.3	0.00	2.6	0.03	0.24	0.1	150.4	0.18	50.0	245.9
47	**Cheese,** Cheddar or American type, natural, 1 slice (1 oz)	28.4	114.1	6.0	29.7	0.00	5.2	0.02	0.23	0.1	204.5	0.19	27.9	175.9
114	**Cheese,** cream, 1 small package (3 oz)	85.0	296.7	18.7	93.2	0.00	11.2	0.04	0.36	0.8	67.9	1.02	101.5	251.2
177	**Cheese,** Mozzarella, 1 slice (1 oz)	28.4	79.4	3.1	15.3	0.00	2.8	0.02	0.26	0.1	207.3	0.07	26.9	149.6
87	**Cheese,** Parmesan, dry grated, 1 tablespoon (0.2 oz)	5.0	22.8	1.0	3.9	0.00	0.4	0.01	0.07	0.0	68.8	0.05	5.4	93.1
157	**Cheese,** Swiss, 1 slice (1 oz)	28.4	106.5	5.0	26.0	0.00	1.8	0.02	0.48	0.1	272.4	0.05	31.4	73.7
196	**Cheeseburger,** 1 Burger King cheeseburger (4.1 oz)	115.0	270.2	4.9	36.8	1.64	67.2	0.14	1.08	1.1	138.0	2.49	245.6	677.8
184	**Chicken** breast, broiled, no bone or skin, 1/2 medium breast (2.9 oz)	81.0	132.5	0.8	68.3	0.00	3.2	0.48	0.27	0.2	12.2	0.84	205.7	321.0
138	**Chicken** breast, roasted, no bone or skin, 1/2 medium breast (3 oz)	86.0	140.7	0.9	72.5	0.00	3.4	0.51	0.29	0.2	13.0	0.89	218.4	340.8
199	**Chicken** noodle soup, 1 cup (8 fl oz)	241.0	74.8	0.6	6.1	0.74	18.6	0.03	0.16	0.1	15.9	0.77	55.2	931.3
139	**Chicken** nuggets, 1 nugget (0.6 oz)	18.0	51.1	1.0	10.8	0.07	5.2	0.06	0.05	0.4	2.9	0.23	44.3	95.8
183	**Chicken or turkey breast,** prepackaged or deli, 1 slice (1 oz)	28.4	31.2	0.1	11.6	0.00	1.1	0.10	0.57	0.1	2.0	0.11	78.8	405.7
60	**Chicken or turkey loaf,** prepackaged or deli, 1 slice (1 oz)	28.4	43.0	0.6	14.0	0.00	1.0	0.08	0.06	0.1	10.9	0.34	70.8	156.8

From the book *Stikky Weight Management*. Rankings are in order of how often items are consumed. www.stikky.com.

SOURCE: 1994-6, 1998 *Continuing Survey of Food Intakes*, USDA, www.barc.usda.gov/bhnrc/foodsurvey/home.htm

Rank		Grams g	Calories kcal	Sat Fat g	Cholesterol mg	Fiber g	Folate mcg	Vitamin B6 mg	Vitamin B12 mcg	Vitamin E ATE	Calcium mg	Iron mg	Potassium mg	Sodium mg
144	**Chicken** patty, fillet or tenders, breaded, cooked, 1 patty (3 oz)	85.0	241.4	4.6	51.0	0.34	24.7	0.26	0.26	1.7	13.6	1.06	209.1	452.2
185	**Chili con carne,** with beans, 1 cup (9 oz)	254.0	320.7	5.0	59.6	7.44	45.1	0.36	1.94	1.8	59.7	3.80	762.1	1311.9
145	**Chili peppers,** hot sauce, 1 McDonald's packet (0.35 fl oz)	10.5	2.1	0.0	0.0	0.20	1.3	0.01	0.00	0.1	0.5	0.04	59.2	2.6
165	**Chocolate,** milk, 1 bar (1.45 oz)	41.0	210.3	7.6	9.0	1.39	3.3	0.02	0.16	0.5	78.3	0.57	157.9	33.6
167	**Chocolate syrup,** thin type, 1 tablespoon (0.5 fl oz)	18.8	41.0	0.1	0.0	0.34	0.8	0.00	0.00	0.0	2.6	0.40	42.1	18.0
85	**Coleslaw,** with dressing, 1 fast food order (3.2 oz)	90.0	132.0	1.8	8.7	1.72	29.2	0.16	0.04	1.8	34.4	0.49	186.5	252.1
159	**Cookie,** butter or sugar cookie, 1 small (2", 0.33 oz)	9.0	42.8	0.6	4.4	0.08	4.3	0.00	0.01	0.2	4.8	0.19	9.3	37.5
63	**Cookie,** chocolate chip, 1 medium (approx 2", 0.35 oz)	10.0	48.1	0.7	0.0	0.25	4.2	0.01	0.00	0.3	2.5	0.28	13.5	31.5
106	**Cookie,** Oreo mini sandwich, 1 (0.1 oz)	2.8	13.2	0.1	0.0	0.09	1.2	0.00	0.00	0.1	0.7	0.11	4.9	16.9
99	**Corn flakes,** Kellogg, 1 cup (1 oz)	28.0	102.2	0.1	0.0	0.78	98.8	0.48	0.00	0.0	1.1	8.68	25.5	297.9
130	**Corn chips or corn-cheese chips,** 10 chips (0.6 oz)	18.0	97.0	0.8	0.0	0.88	3.6	0.04	0.00	0.2	22.9	0.24	25.6	113.4
129	**Corn chips or corn-chesse puffs and twists,** 10 pieces (0.5 oz)	15.0	83.1	1.0	0.6	0.17	18.0	0.02	0.02	0.8	8.7	0.35	24.9	157.5
175	**Corn,** yellow, cooked, 1 cup (5.8 oz)	164.0	132.8	0.3	0.0	3.28	75.7	0.08	0.00	0.2	8.2	1.41	319.8	351.0
171	**Cornbread,** 1 piece (2.3 oz)	65.0	183.2	1.2	26.3	1.54	38.7	0.06	0.10	1.0	130.7	1.57	90.4	318.1
181	**Cracker,** graham, 1 large rectangular piece or 4 small (0.5 oz)	14.0	59.2	0.2	0.0	0.39	8.4	0.01	0.00	0.3	3.4	0.52	18.9	84.7
195	**Cracker,** Ritz Bits sandwich, 1 (0.08 oz)	2.4	11.9	0.1	0.0	0.03	0.6	0.00	0.00	0.0	2.4	0.07	6.2	21.9
52	**Cracker,** saltine, 1 cracker (0.1 oz)	3.0	13.0	0.1	0.0	0.09	3.7	0.00	0.00	0.0	3.6	0.16	3.8	39.1
102	**Cracker,** snack, 1 cracker (0.15 oz)	4.0	20.1	0.2	0.0	0.06	3.1	0.00	0.00	0.2	4.8	0.14	5.3	33.9
55	**Cream,** half and half, 1 individual container (0.5 fl oz)	15.0	19.6	1.1	5.5	0.00	0.4	0.01	0.05	0.1	15.7	0.01	19.4	6.1
126	**Cream substitute,** liquid, 1 individual container (0.5 fl oz)	15.0	20.3	0.3	0.0	0.00	0.0	0.00	0.00	0.2	1.4	0.00	28.6	11.9
33	**Cream substitute,** powdered, 1 packet	3.0	16.4	1.0	0.0	0.00	0.0	0.00	0.00	0.0	0.7	0.03	24.4	5.4
110	**Croutons,** 1 fast food package (0.35 oz)	10.0	46.5	0.5	0.3	0.50	8.8	0.01	0.01	0.2	9.6	0.28	18.1	123.8
37	**Cucumber,** 1 medium (7" long, 7.1 oz)	201.0	24.1	0.1	0.0	1.41	28.1	0.14	0.00	0.2	28.1	0.32	297.5	4.0
179	**Cupcake,** chocolate, with icing or filling, 1 cupcake (2-3/4", 1.6 oz)	46.0	173.0	1.3	7.8	0.37	13.3	0.01	0.06	0.9	33.6	1.55	56.1	195.5
162	**Doughnut,** cake type, 1 medium doughnut (3-1/4", 1.7 oz)	47.0	197.9	1.7	17.4	0.71	22.1	0.03	0.11	1.6	20.7	0.92	59.7	256.6
176	**Doughnut,** raised or yeast, 1 medium doughnut (3-3/4", 2.1 oz)	60.0	241.8	3.5	3.6	0.72	25.8	0.03	0.05	1.7	25.8	1.22	64.8	205.2
182	**Dressing,** French, 1 tablespoon (0.5 fl oz)	15.6	67.0	1.5	0.0	0.00	0.7	0.00	0.02	1.3	1.7	0.06	12.3	213.7
48	**Dressing,** Italian, made with vinegar and oil, 1 tablespoon (0.5 fl oz)	14.7	68.7	1.0	0.0	0.00	0.7	0.00	0.02	1.5	1.5	0.03	2.2	115.7
62	**Dressing,** made with sour cream or buttermilk, 1 tablespoon (0.5 fl oz)	14.7	71.4	1.1	0.7	0.01	0.2	0.00	0.00	1.5	2.1	0.01	4.1	173.6
53	**Dressing,** mayonnaise-type, 1 tablespoon (0.5 fl oz)	14.7	57.3	0.7	3.8	0.00	0.9	0.00	0.03	0.6	2.1	0.03	1.3	104.5
115	**Egg,** whole, boiled, 1 medium (1.5 oz)	44.0	67.9	1.4	185.8	0.00	19.3	0.05	0.49	0.5	22.0	0.52	55.2	122.3
21	**Egg,** whole, fried, 1 medium (1.4 oz)	40.0	78.8	1.7	183.1	0.00	15.2	0.06	0.37	0.7	21.8	0.62	53.0	207.0
80	**Frankfurter or hot dog,** beef, 1 frankfurter (2 oz)	57.0	185.5	7.0	36.3	0.00	2.1	0.04	0.79	0.1	12.1	0.87	95.6	591.0
191	**Frosted Flakes,** Kellogg, 1 cup (1.5 oz)	41.0	157.9	0.1	0.0	0.82	123.0	0.66	0.00	0.1	0.8	5.95	27.1	264.5
70	**Grape,** 1 cup, with seeds (5.4 oz)	154.0	109.3	0.3	0.0	1.54	6.0	0.17	0.00	1.1	16.9	0.40	284.9	3.1
150	**Grapefruit,** 1/2 medium (approx 4", 4.5 oz)	128.0	41.0	0.0	0.0	1.41	13.1	0.05	0.00	0.3	15.4	0.12	177.9	0.0
65	**Gravy,** beef or meat, 1 cup (8 fl oz)	233.0	123.5	2.7	7.0	0.93	4.7	0.02	0.23	0.1	14.0	1.63	188.7	1304.8
152	**Gravy,** poultry, 1 cup (8 fl oz)	238.0	188.0	3.4	4.8	0.95	4.8	0.02	0.24	0.4	47.6	1.12	259.4	1373.3
30	**Ham,** sliced, prepackaged or deli, 1 slice (4-1/4" sq, 0.75 oz)	21.0	34.0	0.6	11.1	0.00	0.6	0.08	0.17	0.1	1.5	0.19	62.4	268.4
158	**Ham,** smoked or cured, 1 medium slice (4-1/2" x 2-1/2" x 1/4", 1.5 oz)	42.0	72.0	1.2	24.4	0.00	1.3	0.14	0.29	0.1	3.4	0.58	161.9	605.9
86	**Hard candy,** 1 piece (0.2 oz)	6.0	22.4	0.0	0.0	0.00	0.0	0.00	0.00	0.0	0.2	0.02	0.3	2.3
116	**Honey,** 1 tablespoon (0.5 fl oz)	21.0	63.8	0.0	0.0	0.04	0.4	0.01	0.00	0.0	1.3	0.09	10.9	0.8
32	**Ice cream,** 1 cup (8 fl oz)	133.0	267.3	9.0	58.5	0.00	6.7	0.06	0.52	0.0	170.2	0.12	264.7	106.4
170	**Ice pop,** 1 single stick (3.1 oz)	88.0	63.4	0.0	0.0	0.00	0.0	0.00	0.00	0.0	0.0	0.00	3.5	10.6
83	**Jam,** preserves, all flavors, 1 tablespoon (0.75 oz)	21.0	50.8	0.0	0.0	0.24	6.9	0.00	0.00	0.0	4.2	0.10	16.2	8.4
31	**Jelly,** all flavors, 1 cup (8 fl oz)	300.0	813.0	0.1	0.0	3.00	3.0	0.06	0.00	0.0	24.0	0.60	192.0	108.0
6	**Lemon,** 1 wedge or slice (1/8 of one 2-1/8" lemon, 0.25 oz)	7.0	2.0	0.0	0.0	0.20	0.7	0.01	0.00	0.0	1.8	0.04	9.7	0.1
160	**Lettuce,** 1 cup, shredded or chopped (1.9 oz)	55.0	6.6	0.0	0.0	0.77	30.8	0.02	0.00	0.2	10.5	0.28	86.9	5.0
160	**Macaroni or noodles with cheese,** 1 cup (8.6 oz)	243.0	476.1	9.9	36.6	1.80	72.8	0.12	0.44	1.7	392.4	2.75	319.7	972.5
107	**Macaroni or noodles with cheese,** made from dry mix, 1 cup (6.75 oz)	191.0	397.2	4.8	8.7	1.97	101.0	0.07	0.19	2.3	148.8	2.04	152.9	749.3
84	**Maple syrup** or cane syrup, 1 tablespoon (0.5 fl oz)	20.0	53.0	0.0	0.0	0.00	0.0	0.00	0.00	0.0	1.0	0.01	1.2	12.2
51	**Margarine,** stick, salted, 1 tablespoon (0.5 oz)	14.2	102.1	2.2	0.0	0.00	0.1	0.00	0.01	1.7	4.3	0.01	6.0	133.9

Rank		Grams	Calories	Sat Fat	Cholesterol	Fiber	Folate	Vitamin B6	Vitamin B12	Vitamin E	Calcium	Iron	Potassium	Sodium
		g	kcal	g	mg	g	mg	mg	mcg	ATE	mg	mg	mg	mg
192	**Margarine,** stick, unsalted, 1 tablespoon (0.5 oz)	14.2	102.1	2.2	0.0	0.00	0.1	0.00	0.01	1.7	2.4	0.00	3.6	0.3
59	**Margarine,** tub, salted, 1 tablespoon (0.5 oz)	14.2	101.7	1.8	0.0	0.00	0.1	0.00	0.01	1.7	3.7	0.00	5.4	153.2
100	**Margarine-like spread,** stick, salted, 1 tablespoon (0.5 oz)	14.3	77.2	1.7	0.0	0.00	0.1	0.00	0.01	1.3	3.0	0.00	4.3	142.1
28	**Margarine-like spread,** tub, salted, 1 tablespoon (0.5 oz)	14.3	77.2	1.4	0.0	0.00	0.1	0.00	0.01	1.3	3.0	0.00	4.3	142.1
19	**Mayonnaise,** regular, 1 salad dressing packet (2 oz)	55.0	394.2	6.5	32.5	0.00	4.2	0.32	0.14	6.5	9.9	0.28	18.7	312.6
178	**Meat loaf** made with beef, 1 medium slice (3.8 oz)	108.0	229.3	4.9	89.1	0.44	16.3	0.14	1.64	0.1	43.1	2.02	293.4	435.4
154	**Muffin,** English, toasted, 1 muffin (1.75 oz)	50.0	127.5	0.1	0.0	1.45	37.0	0.02	0.02	0.1	94.5	1.36	71.5	252.0
146	**Muffin,** fruit and/or nuts, 1 medium muffin (2-3/4", 2 oz)	57.0	157.9	0.8	17.1	1.48	25.7	0.01	0.33	0.6	32.5	0.92	70.1	254.8
15	**Mustard,** 1 packet (0.16 oz)	5.0	3.8	0.0	0.0	0.14	0.4	0.00	0.00	0.1	4.2	0.10	6.5	62.6
27	**Onion,** 1 medium (2-1/2", 3.9 oz)	110.0	41.8	0.0	0.0	1.98	20.9	0.13	0.00	0.1	22.0	0.24	172.7	3.3
43	**Orange,** 1 medium (2-5/8", 4.6 oz)	131.0	61.6	0.0	0.0	3.14	39.7	0.08	0.00	0.3	52.4	0.13	237.1	0.0
76	**Pancake,** plain, 1 medium pancake (5", 1.4 oz)	40.0	91.6	0.3	3.6	0.72	18.0	0.02	0.06	0.3	24.8	1.39	29.2	203.6
128	**Peach,** 1 medium (2-1/2", 3.5 oz)	98.0	42.1	0.0	0.0	1.96	3.3	0.02	0.00	0.7	4.9	0.11	193.1	0.0
35	**Peanut butter,** 1 tablespoon (0.6 oz)	16.0	94.9	1.7	0.0	0.94	11.8	0.07	0.00	1.6	6.1	0.29	107.0	74.7
163	**Pear,** 1 medium pear (5.9 oz)	166.0	97.9	0.0	0.0	3.98	12.1	0.03	0.00	0.8	18.3	0.42	207.5	0.0
132	**Pepper,** sweet, green, 1 medium (2-3/4" long, 2-1/2", 4.2 oz)	119.0	32.1	0.0	0.0	2.14	26.2	0.30	0.00	0.8	10.7	0.55	210.6	2.4
56	**Pickle,** dill, 1 medium (3-3/4" long, 2.3 oz)	65.0	11.7	0.0	0.0	0.78	0.7	0.01	0.00	0.1	5.9	0.34	75.4	833.3
111	**Pizza,** cheese, thin crust, 1 medium pizza (13", 20.8 oz)	590.0	1517.7	24.7	87.6	9.88	272.5	0.52	0.83	8.9	1378.1	12.23	1250.7	3857.5
194	**Pizza with meat and vegetables,** thin crust, 1 medium pizza (13", 26.1 oz)	740.0	1809.1	34.5	148.7	12.60	272.2	0.87	2.21	9.6	1268.4	13.98	1704.3	4768.4
131	**Pizza with meat,** thick crust, 1 medium pizza (13", 26.1 oz)	740.0	2280.1	35.0	134.8	12.31	410.9	0.62	2.01	9.8	1131.3	18.32	1404.9	5049.8
69	**Pizza with meat,** thin crust, 1 medium pizza (13", 23.5 oz)	666.0	1953.2	38.7	168.9	9.86	275.5	0.69	2.52	9.1	1384.6	13.73	1529.4	5106.0
141	**Popcorn,** popped in oil, buttered, 1 cup, popped (0.5 oz)	14.0	72.9	1.3	3.0	1.26	2.2	0.03	0.00	0.0	1.6	0.35	28.8	123.0
188	**Popcorn,** popped in oil, unbuttered, 1 cup, popped (0.4 oz)	11.0	55.0	0.5	0.0	1.10	1.9	0.02	0.00	0.0	1.1	0.31	24.8	97.2
46	**Pork bacon,** smoked or cured, 1 medium slice (0.3 oz cooked)	8.0	46.1	1.4	6.8	0.00	0.4	0.02	0.14	0.0	1.0	0.05	38.9	127.7
103	**Pork sausage,** 1 patty (3-7/8" dia x 1/4" thick raw, 1 oz cooked)	27.0	99.6	2.9	22.4	0.00	0.5	0.09	0.47	0.0	8.6	0.34	97.5	349.4
125	**Potato,** baked, peel eaten, 1 medium (2-1/4" to 3", 4.3 oz)	122.0	132.2	0.0	0.0	2.91	13.3	0.42	0.00	0.1	12.3	1.65	507.0	288.9
79	**Potato,** baked, peel not eaten, 1 medium (2-1/4" to 3")	98.0	90.6	0.0	0.0	1.46	8.9	0.29	0.00	0.0	5.0	0.34	380.9	237.2
198	**Potato,** oiled, without peel, 1 medium (2-1/4" to 3" dia, 4.3 oz)	122.0	104.3	0.0	0.0	2.18	10.8	0.33	0.00	0.1	9.9	0.38	397.8	295.3
25	**Potato,** chips, 1 chip, regular (0.05 oz)	1.4	7.5	0.2	0.0	0.06	0.6	0.01	0.00	0.1	0.3	0.02	17.9	8.3
20	**Potato,** french fries, 1 fast food order (3.5 oz)	100.0	309.1	5.0	0.4	3.20	33.0	0.26	0.12	0.2	16.0	1.35	712.0	163.0
68	**Potato,** french fries, 10 strips (2" to 3-1/2", 1.75 oz)	50.0	140.7	2.0	0.1	1.60	13.9	0.14	0.05	0.1	7.0	0.66	318.8	93.8
108	**Potato,** home fries, 1 medium potato (2-1/4" to 3", 2.5 oz)	70.0	96.8	0.6	0.0	1.17	6.4	0.18	0.00	1.0	4.5	0.20	228.7	162.5
73	**Potato,** mashed from fresh, made with milk and fat, 1 cup (7.4 oz)	210.0	225.8	1.8	2.4	3.07	16.7	0.47	0.11	1.2	51.8	0.55	608.7	658.8
180	**Potato salad,** 1 cup (6.8 oz)	193.0	274.8	2.3	11.0	3.10	21.5	0.55	0.05	2.4	21.0	0.79	594.2	799.6
64	**Pretzel,** hard, 1-3 ring pretzel (0.1 oz)	3.0	11.4	0.0	0.0	0.10	5.1	0.00	0.00	0.0	1.1	0.13	4.4	51.5
189	**Radish,** 1 medium (3/4" to 1", 0.15 oz)	4.5	0.9	0.0	0.0	0.07	1.2	0.00	0.00	0.0	0.9	0.01	10.4	1.1
190	**Raisins,** 50 raisins (0.9 oz)	26.0	78.0	0.0	0.0	1.04	0.9	0.06	0.00	0.2	12.7	0.54	195.3	3.1
164	**Refried beans,** 1 cup (8.9 oz)	253.0	484.8	8.8	20.7	17.57	323.1	0.37	0.00	2.1	108.8	5.23	993.1	665.5
173	**Rice Krispies,** 1 cup (0.9 oz)	26.0	98.0	0.1	0.0	0.29	91.8	0.44	0.00	0.0	2.6	1.56	33.3	278.7
92	**Rice,** white, fat added in cooking, 1 cup cooked (5.75 oz)	163.0	263.5	1.5	0.0	0.61	88.5	0.14	0.01	1.2	18.3	1.84	57.3	648.1
44	**Rice,** white, fat not added in cooking, 1 cup cooked (5.6 oz)	158.0	203.5	0.1	0.0	0.63	90.8	0.15	0.00	0.1	16.0	1.88	54.9	577.5
187	**Salami,** 1 slice (4" dia x 1/8" thick, 0.8 oz)	23.0	57.5	1.9	15.0	0.00	0.5	0.05	0.84	0.1	3.0	0.61	45.5	245.0
75	**Salsa,** red, cooked, not homemade, 1 tablespoon (0.5 fl oz)	16.0	3.5	0.0	0.0	0.30	2.2	0.02	0.00	0.1	7.4	0.12	29.6	41.4
155	**Soup,** mostly noodles, 1 cup (8 fl oz)	233.0	157.6	1.7	0.2	1.19	3.2	0.01	0.00	2.4	13.4	0.40	50.4	823.1
121	**Sour cream,** 1 cup (8 fl oz)	230.0	492.8	30.0	102.1	0.00	24.8	0.04	0.69	1.3	267.7	0.14	331.2	122.6
193	**Soy sauce,** 1 tablespoon (0.5 fl oz)	16.0	8.5	0.0	0.0	0.13	2.5	0.03	0.00	0.0	2.7	0.32	28.8	914.4
93	**Spaghetti,** plain, fat not added in cooking, 1 cup, cooked (4.9 oz)	140.0	196.2	0.1	0.0	2.37	97.4	0.05	0.00	0.1	9.9	1.95	43.2	325.0
140	**Spaghetti with tomato sauce and meatballs or meat sauce,** 1 cup (8.8 oz)	248.0	323.4	3.2	68.3	3.64	76.0	0.35	1.01	2.1	129.6	3.72	650.4	1075.8
113	**Spaghetti sauce,** 1 cup (8.8 oz)	250.0	142.5	0.7	0.0	4.00	25.0	0.29	0.00	3.1	55.0	1.80	737.5	1030.0
142	**Spaghetti sauce** with beef, homemade-style, 1 cup (8.8 oz)	249.0	287.7	4.5	46.6	4.20	29.8	0.54	1.44	5.3	59.0	3.53	1100.0	1177.4
89	**Strawberries,** 1 cup, whole (5.1 oz)	144.0	43.2	0.0	0.0	3.31	25.5	0.08	0.00	0.2	20.2	0.55	239.0	1.4
58	**Sugar substitute,** aspartame-based, dry powder, 1 individual packet	1.0	3.5	0.0	0.0	0.00	0.0	0.00	0.00	0.0	0.0	0.00	0.0	0.0

Rank		Grams	Calories	Sat Fat	Cholesterol	Fiber	Folate	Vitamin B6	Vitamin B12	Vitamin E	Calcium	Iron	Potassium	Sodium
		g	kcal	g	mg	g	mg	mg	mcg	ATE	mg	mg	mg	mg
36	**Sugar substitute,** saccharin-based, dry powder, 1 individual packet	1.0	**3.6**	0.0	0.0	0.00	0.0	0.00	0.00	0.0	0.0	0.00	45.0	4.0
5	**Sugar,** white, granulated or lump, 1 teaspoon (0.15 oz)	4.2	**16.3**	0.0	0.0	0.00	0.0	0.00	0.00	0.0	0.0	0.00	0.1	0.0
156	**Tart,** breakfast, 1 Pop Tart (1.8 oz)	52.0	**204.4**	0.8	0.0	1.09	33.8	0.20	0.03	1.0	13.5	1.81	58.2	217.9
7	**Tomato,** raw, 1 medium whole (2-3/5", 4.3 oz)	123.0	**25.8**	0.1	0.0	1.35	18.5	0.10	0.00	0.5	6.2	0.55	273.1	11.1
11	**Tomato catsup,** 1 tablespoon (0.5 oz)	15.0	**15.6**	0.0	0.0	0.20	2.3	0.03	0.00	0.2	2.9	0.11	72.2	177.9
45	**Tortilla chips,** 10 chips (0.6 oz)	18.0	**90.2**	0.9	0.0	1.17	1.8	0.05	0.00	0.2	27.7	0.27	35.5	95.0
97	**Tortilla, corn,** 1 medium tortilla (approx 6", 0.7 oz)	19.0	**42.2**	0.1	0.0	0.99	21.7	0.04	0.00	0.0	33.3	0.27	29.3	30.6
133	**Tuna salad,** 1 cup (7.3 oz)	208.0	**295.6**	1.7	41.4	0.96	14.7	0.44	3.43	1.9	27.5	2.15	351.9	853.5
119	**Waffle,** plain, 1 square waffle (4" square, 1.3 oz)	37.0	**97.7**	0.5	8.9	0.85	16.7	0.33	0.93	0.3	85.8	1.65	47.4	291.2
109	**Water** as an ingredient, 1 cup (8 fl oz)	237.0	**0.0**	0.0	0.0	0.00	0.0	0.00	0.00	0.0	4.7	0.02	0.0	7.1
98	**Watermelon,** 1 wedge (1/16 of melon, 10 oz)	286.0	**91.5**	0.1	0.0	1.43	6.3	0.41	0.00	0.4	22.9	0.49	331.8	5.7

Drinks

Rank		Grams	Calories	Sat Fat	Cholesterol	Fiber	Folate	Vitamin B6	Vitamin B12	Vitamin E	Calcium	Iron	Potassium	Sodium
72	**Apple juice,** 1 cup (8 fl oz)	248.0	**116.6**	0.0	0.0	0.25	0.2	0.07	0.00	0.0	17.4	0.92	295.1	7.4
40	**Beer,** 1 can or bottle (12 fl oz)	360.0	**147.6**	0.0	0.0	0.72	21.6	0.18	0.07	0.0	18.0	0.11	90.0	18.0
71	**Beer, lite,** 1 can or bottle (12 fl oz)	360.0	**100.8**	0.0	0.0	0.00	14.8	0.12	0.04	0.0	18.0	0.14	64.8	10.8
34	**Coffee,** regular, from powdered instant, 1 coffee cup (6 fl oz)	179.0	**3.9**	0.0	0.0	0.00	0.0	0.00	0.00	0.0	5.8	0.09	57.7	5.9
1	**Coffee,** regular, ground, 1 coffee cup (6 fl oz)	177.0	**3.5**	0.0	0.0	0.00	0.2	0.00	0.00	0.0	3.5	0.09	95.6	3.5
81	**Coffee,** decaffeinated, from powdered instant, 1 coffee cup (6 fl oz)	179.0	**3.7**	0.0	0.0	0.00	0.0	0.00	0.00	0.0	5.8	0.08	57.2	5.7
41	**Coffee,** decaffeinated, ground, 1 coffee cup (6 fl oz)	177.0	**3.5**	0.0	0.0	0.00	0.0	0.00	0.00	0.0	3.5	0.09	95.6	3.5
2	**Cola-type soft drink,** 1 can (12 fl oz)	369.0	**151.3**	0.0	0.0	0.00	0.0	0.00	0.00	0.0	11.1	0.11	3.7	14.8
137	**Cola-type soft drink,** decaffeinated, 1 can (12 fl oz)	369.0	**151.3**	0.0	0.0	0.00	0.0	0.00	0.00	0.0	11.1	0.11	3.7	14.8
61	**Cola-type soft drink,** decaffeinated, sugar-free, 1 can (12 fl oz)	355.0	**3.6**	0.0	0.0	0.00	0.0	0.00	0.00	0.0	14.2	0.11	0.0	21.3
16	**Cola-type soft drink,** sugar-free, 1 can (12 fl oz)	355.0	**3.6**	0.0	0.0	0.00	0.0	0.00	0.00	0.0	14.2	0.11	0.0	21.3
151	**Cranberry juice** drink with vitamin C added, 1 cup (8 fl oz)	253.0	**144.2**	0.0	0.0	0.25	0.5	0.05	0.00	0.0	7.6	0.38	45.5	5.1
78	**Fruit drink,** 1 cup (8 fl oz)	248.0	**116.6**	0.0	0.0	0.25	2.5	0.00	0.00	0.0	19.8	0.52	62.0	54.6
105	**Fruit punch,** fruit drink, or fruitade, with vitamin C added, 1 cup (8 fl oz)	247.0	**116.1**	0.0	0.0	0.25	3.2	0.00	0.00	0.0	19.8	0.52	61.8	54.3
101	**Fruit-flavored drink,** from sweetened powdered mix, 1 cup (8 fl oz)	250.0	**87.8**	0.0	0.0	0.02	0.2	0.00	0.00	0.0	37.2	0.14	1.2	34.4
67	**Fruit-flavored drink,** from unsweetened powdered mix, 1 cup (8 fl oz)	240.0	**89.7**	0.0	0.0	0.00	0.2	0.00	0.00	0.0	14.1	0.04	0.5	12.5
22	**Fruit-flavored soft drink,** caffeine free, 1 can (12 fl oz)	368.0	**147.2**	0.0	0.0	0.00	0.0	0.00	0.00	0.0	7.4	0.26	3.7	40.5
49	**Fruit-flavored soft drink,** containing caffeine, 1 can (12 fl oz)	372.0	**148.8**	0.0	0.0	0.00	0.0	0.00	0.00	0.0	7.4	0.26	3.7	40.9
143	**Fruit-flavored soft drink,** sugar free, caffeine free, 1 can (12 fl oz)	355.0	**0.0**	0.0	0.0	0.00	0.0	0.00	0.00	0.0	14.2	0.14	7.1	21.3
172	**Fruit-flavored thirst quencher** beverage, 1 cup (8 fl oz)	240.0	**60.0**	0.0	0.0	0.00	0.0	0.00	0.00	0.0	0.0	0.12	26.4	96.0
118	**Lemonade,** 1 Snapple bottle (16 fl oz)	496.0	**198.7**	0.0	0.0	0.44	11.0	0.03	0.00	0.0	15.4	0.83	73.6	16.0
18	**Milk,** 1% fat, 1 cup (8 fl oz)	244.0	**102.1**	1.6	9.8	0.00	12.4	0.10	0.90	0.1	300.1	0.12	380.9	123.2
3	**Milk,** 2% fat, 1 cup (8 fl oz)	244.0	**121.2**	2.9	18.3	0.00	12.4	0.10	0.89	0.2	296.7	0.12	376.7	121.8
10	**Milk,** skim or nonfat, 0.5% or less butterfat, 1 cup (8 fl oz)	245.0	**85.5**	0.3	4.4	0.00	12.7	0.10	0.93	0.1	302.3	0.10	405.7	126.2
4	**Milk,** whole, 1 cup (8 fl oz)	244.0	**149.9**	5.1	33.2	0.00	12.2	0.10	0.87	0.2	291.3	0.12	369.7	119.6
149	**Milk, chocolate,** reduced fat, 1 cup (8 fl oz)	250.0	**178.8**	3.1	17.0	1.25	12.0	0.10	0.85	0.1	284.0	0.60	422.0	150.5
127	**Orange breakfast drink,** 1 cup (8 fl oz)	250.0	**110.0**	0.0	0.0	0.00	20.0	0.03	0.00	0.0	10.0	0.10	102.5	160.0
13	**Orange juice,** unsweetened, 1 cup (8 fl oz)	249.0	**104.6**	0.0	0.0	0.50	45.1	0.22	0.00	0.2	19.9	1.10	435.8	5.0
42	**Orange juice,** frozen, unsweetened (with water), 1 cup (8 fl oz)	249.0	**113.0**	0.0	0.0	0.57	110.4	0.11	0.00	0.2	26.3	0.27	479.0	7.5
134	**Root beer,** 1 can (12 fl oz)	370.0	**151.7**	0.0	0.0	0.00	0.0	0.00	0.00	0.0	18.5	0.19	3.7	48.1
50	**Soft drink,** pepper-type, 1 can (12 fl oz)	369.0	**151.3**	0.0	0.0	0.00	0.0	0.00	0.00	0.0	11.1	0.11	3.7	14.8
153	**Tea,** herbal, 1 teacup (6 fl oz)	178.0	**1.8**	0.0	0.0	0.00	1.1	0.00	0.00	0.0	3.6	0.14	16.0	1.8
148	**Tea,** leaf, decaffeinated, unsweetened, 1 teacup (6 fl oz)	178.0	**1.8**	0.0	0.0	0.00	8.9	0.00	0.00	0.0	0.0	0.04	65.9	5.3
39	**Tea,** leaf, presweetened, 1 fl oz	29.6	**6.0**	0.0	0.0	0.00	1.5	0.00	0.00	0.0	0.0	0.01	10.4	0.9
14	**Tea,** leaf, unsweetened, 1 teacup (6 fl oz)	178.0	**1.8**	0.0	0.0	0.00	9.3	0.00	0.00	0.0	0.0	0.04	65.9	5.3
166	**Tea,** made from powdered instant, presweetened, 1 teacup (6 fl oz)	178.0	**17.5**	0.0	0.0	0.02	0.7	0.01	0.00	0.0	3.9	0.05	45.1	6.1
74	**Wine,** table, dry, 1 wine glass (3.5 fl oz)	103.0	**72.1**	0.0	0.0	0.00	1.1	0.02	0.01	0.0	8.2	0.42	91.7	8.2

Food measurements:

1 ounce (oz) = 28.35 grams (g)
1 fluid ounce (fl oz) = 29.6 milliliters (ml)
1 pound = 16 oz (453.6g)

1 tablespoon = 3 teaspoons = 1/2 fl oz (14.8 ml)
1 cup = 8 fl oz (236.6 ml)
1 pint = 16 fl oz (473.2 ml)

1 kg (1000g) = 35.3 oz
1 liter (1000 ml) = 33.8 fl oz

America's 200 Most Commonly Eaten Foods

Rank		Grams	Calories	Sat Fat	Cholesterol	Fiber	Folate	Vitamin B6	Vitamin B12	Vitamin E	Calcium	Iron	Potassium	Sodium
		g	kcal	g	mg	g	mg	mg	mcg	ATE	mg	mg	mg	mg
17	**Apple**, raw, 1 medium large (2-3/4", 4.9 oz)	138.0	81.4	0.1	0.0	3.73	3.9	0.07	0.00	0.4	9.7	0.25	158.7	0.0
169	**Bacon**, 1 medium slice (0.3 oz cooked)	8.0	46.1	1.4	6.8	0.00	0.4	0.02	0.14	0.0	1.0	0.13	38.9	127.7
123	**Bagel**, 1 medium (2-3/4" to 3-1/4", 2 oz)	57.0	156.8	0.1	0.0	1.31	50.2	0.03	0.00	0.0	42.2	2.03	57.6	304.4
94	**Bagel**, toasted, 1 medium (2-3/4" to 3-1/4", 1.9 oz)	53.0	156.4	0.1	0.0	1.33	39.8	0.03	0.00	0.0	42.4	2.02	57.8	304.2
12	**Banana**, 1 medium (7" to 7-7/8" long, 4.2 oz)	118.0	108.6	0.2	0.0	2.83	22.5	0.68	0.00	0.3	7.1	0.37	467.3	1.2
91	**Barbecue sauce**, 1 packet (0.3 fl oz)	9.3	7.0	0.0	0.0	0.11	0.4	0.01	0.00	0.1	1.8	0.08	16.2	75.8
117	**Beans**, green, 10 beans (2.2 oz)	62.0	12.4	0.0	0.0	1.18	18.7	0.02	0.00	0.1	16.1	0.56	61.6	162.4
104	**Beef**, ground, lean, 1 medium patty (4 oz, raw, 3.1 oz cooked)	88.0	237.4	6.3	75.9	0.00	7.9	0.23	2.05	0.2	9.8	1.84	262.7	351.3
57	**Beef**, ground, regular, 1 medium patty (4 oz, raw, 3 oz cooked)	85.0	243.6	6.9	75.9	0.00	7.6	0.23	2.47	0.2	9.4	2.06	246.2	344.4
95	**Beef**, patty, 1 medium patty (4 oz, raw, 3 oz cooked)	85.0	232.1	6.3	73.8	0.00	7.6	0.22	2.15	0.2	8.7	1.94	253.0	340.1
124	**Beef**, roasted, lean only, 1 medium slice (4-1/2" x 2-1/2" x 1/4", 1.5 oz)	42.0	82.9	1.4	32.3	0.00	3.4	0.14	1.07	0.1	2.6	1.08	158.0	96.1
82	**Beef steak**, broiled or baked, lean only, 1 medium steak (5.5 oz cooked)	156.0	307.5	4.7	125.1	0.00	14.4	0.71	3.93	0.2	13.8	4.27	636.4	605.2
122	**Biscuit**, baking powder or buttermilk type, 1 regular biscuit (0.7 oz)	19.0	65.7	0.7	0.0	0.30	8.2	0.01	0.00	0.3	3.8	0.49	29.8	228.4
168	**Biscuit**, McDonald's, 1 biscuit (2.5 oz)	72.0	262.1	1.8	0.7	0.94	42.5	0.03	0.10	2.1	35.3	2.38	161.3	757.4
136	**Bologna**, 1 medium slice (4-1/2" dia x 1/8" thick, 1 oz)	28.4	89.6	3.0	15.6	0.00	1.4	0.05	0.38	0.1	3.4	0.43	51.0	288.9
186	**Bread**, French or Vienna, 1 medium slice (4-3/4" x 4" x 1/2", 0.9 oz)	25.0	68.5	0.2	0.0	0.75	23.8	0.01	0.00	0.1	18.8	0.63	28.3	152.3
161	**Bread**, Italian, Grecian, Armenian, 1 medium slice (0.7 oz)	20.0	54.2	0.2	0.0	0.54	19.0	0.01	0.00	0.1	15.6	0.59	22.0	116.8
147	**Bread**, rye, 1 regular slice (0.9 oz)	26.0	67.3	0.2	0.0	1.51	22.4	0.02	0.00	0.1	19.0	0.74	43.2	171.6
8	**Bread**, white, 1 regular slice (0.9 oz)	26.0	69.4	0.1	0.3	0.60	24.7	0.02	0.01	0.1	28.1	0.79	30.9	139.9
23	**Bread**, white, toasted, 1 regular slice (0.8 oz)	23.0	67.4	0.1	0.2	0.58	15.8	0.01	0.00	0.1	27.4	0.77	30.1	136.2
38	**Bread**, whole wheat, 100%, 1 regular slice (1 oz)	28.0	68.9	0.3	0.0	1.93	14.0	0.05	0.00	0.3	20.2	0.92	70.6	147.6
77	**Bread**, whole wheat, 100%, toasted, 1 regular slice (0.9 oz)	25.0	69.3	0.3	0.0	1.85	9.8	0.05	0.00	0.3	20.3	0.93	70.8	148.0
135	**Bread**, whole wheat, other than 100%, 1 regular slice (0.9 oz)	26.0	67.6	0.2	0.0	1.12	20.0	0.03	0.00	0.1	27.3	0.86	52.3	137.8
200	**Bread**, whole wheat, other than 100%, toasted, 1 regular slice (0.9 oz)	24.0	67.7	0.2	0.0	1.27	15.6	0.02	0.00	0.1	27.4	0.86	52.3	138.2
112	**Bread, roll**, hoagie, submarine, 1 medium (8" long, 3.3 oz)	94.0	268.8	1.1	0.0	2.54	119.4	0.04	0.06	1.5	130.7	2.98	132.5	526.4
197	**Bread, roll**, sweet, cinnamon bun, frosted, 1 medium (2" - 2-1/2", 1.9 oz)	55.0	208.5	1.6	29.1	1.06	22.9	0.05	0.06	1.4	33.1	0.71	50.9	193.8
9	**Bread, roll**, white, soft, 1 large hamburger, frankfurter, onion roll (1.5 oz)	43.0	123.0	0.5	0.0	1.16	54.6	0.02	0.03	0.7	59.8	1.36	60.6	240.8
174	**Broccoli**, cooked, from fresh, 1 cup flowerets (3.4 oz)	97.0	27.0	0.1	0.0	2.80	48.2	0.14	0.00	1.6	44.5	0.81	281.6	255.0
29	**Butter**, stick, salted, 1 tablespoon (0.5 oz)	14.2	101.8	7.2	31.1	0.00	0.4	0.00	0.02	0.2	3.4	0.02	3.7	117.3
96	**Butter**, stick, unsalted, 1 tablespoon (0.5 oz)	14.2	101.8	7.2	31.1	0.00	0.4	0.00	0.02	0.2	3.3	0.02	3.7	1.6
66	**Cantaloupe** (muskmelon), 1 wedge (1/8 of medium melon, 2.4 oz)	69.0	24.2	0.0	0.0	0.55	11.7	0.08	0.00	0.1	7.6	0.14	213.2	6.2
26	**Carrot**, raw, 1 small (5-1/2" long, 1.75 oz)	50.0	21.5	0.0	0.0	1.50	7.0	0.07	0.00	0.2	13.5	0.25	161.5	17.5
88	**Celery**, 1 medium stalk (7-1/2" - 8" long) (1.4 oz)	40.0	6.4	0.0	0.0	0.68	11.2	0.03	0.00	0.1	16.0	0.16	114.8	34.8
90	**Cheerios**, 1 cup (1.1 oz)	30.0	109.5	0.4	0.0	2.64	99.9	0.50	0.00	0.2	55.2	8.10	88.5	284.1
24	**Cheese**, Cheddar or American type, processed, 1 slice (1 oz)	28.4	95.0	4.6	19.4	0.00	2.1	0.04	0.30	0.2	164.5	0.22	74.4	346.9
54	**Cheese**, Cheddar or American type, 1 slice (0.85 oz)	24.0	85.7	4.3	19.3	0.00	2.6	0.03	0.24	0.1	150.4	0.18	50.0	245.9
47	**Cheese**, Cheddar or American type, natural, 1 slice (1 oz)	28.4	114.1	6.0	29.7	0.00	5.2	0.02	0.23	0.1	204.5	0.19	27.9	175.9
114	**Cheese**, cream, 1 small package (3 oz)	85.0	296.7	18.7	93.2	0.00	11.2	0.04	0.36	0.8	67.9	1.02	101.5	251.2
177	**Cheese**, Mozzarella, 1 slice (1 oz)	28.4	79.4	3.1	15.3	0.00	2.8	0.02	0.26	0.1	207.3	0.07	26.9	149.6
87	**Cheese**, Parmesan, dry grated, 1 tablespoon (0.2 oz)	5.0	22.8	1.0	3.9	0.00	0.4	0.01	0.07	0.0	68.8	0.05	5.4	93.1
157	**Cheese**, Swiss, 1 slice (1 oz)	28.4	106.5	5.0	26.0	0.00	1.8	0.02	0.48	0.1	272.4	0.05	31.4	73.7
196	**Cheeseburger**, 1 Burger King cheeseburger (4.1 oz)	115.0	270.2	4.9	36.3	1.64	67.2	0.14	1.08	1.1	138.0	2.49	245.6	677.8
184	**Chicken** breast, broiled, no bone or skin, 1/2 medium breast (2.9 oz)	81.0	132.5	0.8	68.3	0.00	3.2	0.48	0.27	0.2	12.2	0.84	205.7	321.0
138	**Chicken** breast, roasted, no bone or skin, 1/2 medium breast (3 oz)	86.0	140.7	0.9	72.5	0.00	3.4	0.51	0.29	0.2	13.0	0.89	218.4	340.8
199	**Chicken** noodle soup, 1 cup (8 fl oz)	241.0	74.8	0.6	6.1	0.74	18.6	0.03	0.16	0.1	15.9	0.77	55.2	931.3
139	**Chicken** nuggets, 1 nugget (0.6 oz)	18.0	51.1	1.0	10.8	0.07	5.2	0.06	0.05	0.4	2.9	0.23	44.3	95.8
183	**Chicken or turkey breast**, prepackaged or deli, 1 slice (1 oz)	28.4	31.2	0.1	11.6	0.00	1.1	0.10	0.57	0.0	2.0	0.11	78.8	405.7
60	**Chicken or turkey loaf**, prepackaged or deli, 1 slice (1 oz)	28.4	43.0	0.6	14.0	0.00	1.0	0.08	0.26	0.1	10.9	0.34	70.8	156.8

Rank		Grams g	Calories kcal	Sat Fat g	Cholesterol mg	Fiber g	Folate mg	Vitamin B6 mg	Vitamin B12 mcg	Vitamin E ATE	Calcium mg	Iron mg	Potassium mg	Sodium mg
144	**Chicken** patty, fillet or tenders, breaded, cooked, 1 patty (3 oz)	85.0	241.4	4.6	51.0	0.34	24.7	0.26	0.26	1.7	13.6	1.06	209.1	452.2
185	**Chili con carne**, with beans, 1 cup (9 oz)	254.0	320.7	5.0	59.6	7.44	45.1	0.36	1.94	1.8	59.7	3.80	762.1	1311.9
145	**Chili peppers**, hot sauce, 1 McDonald's packet (0.35 fl oz)	10.5	2.1	0.0	0.0	0.20	1.3	0.01	0.00	0.1	0.5	0.04	59.2	2.6
165	**Chocolate**, milk, 1 bar (1.45 oz)	41.0	210.3	7.6	9.0	1.39	3.3	0.02	0.16	0.5	78.3	0.57	157.9	33.6
167	**Chocolate syrup**, thin type, 1 tablespoon (0.5 fl oz)	18.8	41.0	0.1	0.0	0.34	0.8	0.00	0.00	0.0	2.6	0.40	42.1	18.0
85	**Coleslaw**, with dressing, 1 fast food order (3.2 oz)	90.0	132.0	1.8	8.7	1.72	29.2	0.16	0.04	1.8	34.4	0.49	186.5	252.1
159	**Cookie**, butter or sugar cookie, 1 small (2", 0.33 oz)	9.0	42.8	0.6	4.4	0.08	4.3	0.00	0.01	0.2	4.8	0.19	9.3	37.5
63	**Cookie**, chocolate chip, 1 medium (approx 2", 0.35 oz)	10.0	48.1	0.7	0.0	0.25	4.2	0.01	0.00	0.3	2.5	0.28	13.5	31.5
106	**Cookie**, Oreo mini sandwich, 1 (0.1 oz)	2.8	13.2	0.1	0.0	0.09	1.2	0.00	0.00	0.1	0.7	0.11	4.9	16.9
99	**Corn flakes**, Kellogg, 1 cup (1 oz)	28.0	102.2	0.1	0.0	0.78	98.8	0.48	0.00	0.0	1.1	8.68	25.5	297.9
130	**Corn chips or corn-cheese chips**, 10 chips (0.6 oz)	18.0	97.0	0.8	0.0	0.88	3.6	0.04	0.00	0.2	22.9	0.24	25.6	113.4
129	**Corn chips or corn-cheese puffs and twists**, 10 pieces (0.5 oz)	15.0	83.1	1.0	0.6	0.17	18.0	0.02	0.02	0.8	8.7	0.35	24.9	157.5
175	**Corn**, yellow, cooked, 1 cup (5.8 oz)	164.0	132.8	0.3	0.0	3.28	75.7	0.08	0.00	0.2	8.2	1.41	319.8	351.0
171	**Cornbread**, 1 piece (2.3 oz)	65.0	183.2	1.2	26.3	1.54	38.7	0.06	0.10	1.0	130.7	1.57	90.4	318.1
181	**Cracker**, graham, 1 large rectangular piece or 4 small (0.5 oz)	14.0	59.2	0.2	0.0	0.39	8.4	0.01	0.00	0.3	3.4	0.52	18.9	84.7
195	**Cracker**, Ritz Bits sandwich, 1 (0.08 oz)	2.4	11.9	0.1	0.0	0.03	0.6	0.00	0.00	0.0	2.4	0.07	6.2	21.9
52	**Cracker**, saltine, 1 cracker (0.1 oz)	3.0	13.0	0.1	0.0	0.09	3.7	0.00	0.00	0.0	3.6	0.16	3.8	39.1
102	**Cracker**, snack, 1 cracker (0.15 oz)	4.0	20.1	0.2	0.0	0.06	3.1	0.00	0.00	0.2	4.8	0.14	5.3	33.9
55	**Cream**, half and half, 1 individual container (0.5 fl oz)	15.0	19.6	1.1	5.5	0.00	0.4	0.01	0.05	0.1	15.7	0.01	19.4	6.1
126	**Cream substitute**, liquid, 1 individual container (0.5 fl oz)	15.0	20.3	0.3	0.0	0.00	0.0	0.00	0.00	0.2	1.4	0.00	28.6	11.9
33	**Cream substitute**, powdered, 1 packet	3.0	16.4	1.0	0.0	0.00	0.0	0.00	0.00	0.0	0.7	0.03	24.4	5.4
110	**Croutons**, 1 fast food package (0.35 oz)	10.0	46.5	0.5	0.3	0.50	8.8	0.01	0.01	0.1	9.6	0.28	18.1	123.8
37	**Cucumber**, 1 medium (7" long, 7.1 oz)	201.0	24.1	0.1	0.0	1.41	28.1	0.14	0.00	0.2	28.1	0.32	297.5	4.0
179	**Cupcake**, chocolate, with icing or filling, 1 cupcake (2-3/4", 1.6 oz)	46.0	173.0	1.3	7.8	0.37	13.3	0.01	0.06	0.9	33.6	1.55	56.1	195.5
162	**Doughnut**, cake type, 1 medium doughnut (3-1/4", 1.7 oz)	47.0	197.9	1.7	17.4	0.71	22.1	0.03	0.11	1.6	20.7	0.92	59.7	256.6
176	**Doughnut**, raised or yeast, 1 medium doughnut (3-3/4", 2.1 oz)	60.0	241.8	3.5	3.6	0.72	25.8	0.03	0.05	1.7	25.8	1.22	64.8	205.2
182	**Dressing**, French, 1 tablespoon (0.5 fl oz)	15.6	67.0	1.5	0.0	0.00	0.7	0.00	0.02	1.3	1.7	0.06	12.3	213.7
48	**Dressing**, Italian, made with vinegar and oil, 1 tablespoon (0.5 fl oz)	14.7	68.7	1.0	0.0	0.00	0.7	0.00	0.02	1.5	1.5	0.03	2.2	115.7
62	**Dressing**, made with sour cream or buttermilk, 1 tablespoon (0.5 fl oz)	14.7	71.4	1.1	0.7	0.01	0.2	0.00	0.00	1.5	2.1	0.01	4.1	173.6
53	**Dressing**, mayonnaise-type, 1 tablespoon (0.5 fl oz)	14.7	57.3	0.7	3.8	0.00	0.9	0.00	0.03	0.6	2.1	0.03	1.3	104.5
115	**Egg**, whole, boiled, 1 medium (1.5 oz)	44.0	67.9	1.4	185.8	0.00	19.3	0.05	0.49	0.5	22.0	0.52	55.2	122.3
21	**Egg**, whole, fried, 1 medium (1.4 oz)	40.0	78.8	1.7	183.1	0.00	15.2	0.06	0.37	0.7	21.8	0.62	53.0	207.0
80	**Frankfurter or hot dog**, beef, 1 frankfurter (2 oz)	57.0	185.5	7.0	36.3	0.00	2.1	0.06	0.79	0.1	12.1	0.87	95.6	591.0
191	**Frosted Flakes**, Kellogg, 1 cup (1.5 oz)	41.0	157.9	0.1	0.0	0.82	123.0	0.66	0.00	0.1	0.8	5.95	27.1	264.5
70	**Grape**, 1 cup, with seeds (5.4 oz)	154.0	109.3	0.3	0.0	1.54	6.0	0.17	0.00	1.1	16.9	0.40	284.9	3.1
150	**Grapefruit**, 1/2 medium (approx 4", 4.5 oz)	128.0	41.0	0.0	0.0	1.41	13.1	0.05	0.00	0.3	15.4	0.12	177.9	0.0
65	**Gravy**, beef or meat, 1 cup (8 fl oz)	233.0	123.5	2.7	7.0	0.93	4.7	0.02	0.23	0.1	14.0	1.63	188.7	1304.8
152	**Gravy**, poultry, 1 cup (8 fl oz)	238.0	188.0	3.4	4.8	0.95	4.8	0.02	0.24	0.4	47.6	1.12	259.4	1373.3
30	**Ham**, sliced, prepackaged or deli, 1 slice (4-1/4" sq, 0.75 oz)	21.0	34.0	0.6	11.1	0.00	0.6	0.08	0.17	0.1	1.5	0.19	62.4	268.4
158	**Ham**, smoked or cured, 1 medium slice (4-1/2" x 2-1/2" x 1/4", 1.5 oz)	42.0	72.0	1.2	24.4	0.00	1.3	0.14	0.29	0.1	3.4	0.58	161.9	605.9
86	**Hard candy**, 1 piece (0.2 oz)	6.0	22.4	0.0	0.0	0.00	0.0	0.00	0.00	0.0	0.2	0.02	0.3	2.3
116	**Honey**, 1 tablespoon (0.5 fl oz)	21.0	63.8	0.0	0.0	0.04	0.4	0.01	0.00	0.0	1.3	0.09	10.9	0.8
32	**Ice cream**, 1 cup (8 fl oz)	133.0	267.3	9.0	58.5	0.00	6.7	0.06	0.52	0.0	170.2	0.12	264.7	106.4
170	**Ice pop**, 1 single stick (3.1 oz)	88.0	63.4	0.0	0.0	0.00	0.0	0.00	0.00	0.0	0.0	0.00	3.5	10.6
83	**Jam**, preserves, all flavors, 1 tablespoon (0.75 oz)	21.0	50.8	0.0	0.0	0.24	6.9	0.00	0.00	0.0	4.2	0.10	16.2	8.4
31	**Jelly**, all flavors, 1 cup (8 fl oz)	300.0	813.0	0.1	0.0	3.00	3.0	0.06	0.00	0.0	24.0	0.60	192.0	108.0
120	**Lemon**, 1 wedge or slice (1/8 of one 2-1/8" lemon, 0.25 oz)	7.0	2.0	0.0	0.0	0.20	0.7	0.01	0.00	0.0	1.8	0.04	9.7	0.1
6	**Lettuce**, 1 cup, shredded or chopped (1.9 oz)	55.0	6.6	0.0	0.0	0.77	30.8	0.02	0.00	0.2	10.5	0.28	86.9	5.0
160	**Macaroni or noodles with cheese**, 1 cup (8.6 oz)	243.0	476.1	9.9	36.6	1.80	72.8	0.12	0.44	1.7	392.4	2.75	319.7	972.5
107	**Macaroni or noodles with cheese**, made from dry mix, 1 cup (6.75 oz)	191.0	397.2	4.8	8.7	1.97	101.0	0.07	0.19	2.3	148.8	2.04	152.9	749.3
84	**Maple syrup** or cane syrup, 1 tablespoon (0.5 fl oz)	20.0	53.0	0.0	0.0	0.00	0.0	0.00	0.00	0.0	1.0	0.01	1.2	12.2
51	**Margarine**, stick, salted, 1 tablespoon (0.5 oz)	14.2	102.1	2.2	0.0	0.00	0.1	0.00	0.01	1.7	4.3	0.01	6.0	133.9

Rank		Grams	Calories	Sat Fat	Cholesterol	Fiber	Folate	Vitamin B6	Vitamin B12	Vitamin E	Calcium	Iron	Potassium	Sodium
		g	kcal	g	mg	g	mg	mg	mcg	ATE	mg	mg	mg	mg
192	**Margarine**, stick, unsalted, 1 tablespoon (0.5 oz)	14.2	102.1	2.2	0.00	0.00	0.1	0.00	0.01	1.7	2.4	0.00	3.6	0.3
59	**Margarine**, tub, salted, 1 tablespoon (0.5 oz)	14.2	101.7	1.8	0.0	0.00	0.1	0.00	0.01	1.7	3.7	0.00	5.4	153.2
100	**Margarine-like spread**, stick, salted, 1 tablespoon (0.5 oz)	14.3	77.2	1.7	0.0	0.00	0.1	0.00	0.01	1.3	3.0	0.00	4.3	142.1
28	**Margarine-like spread**, tub, salted, 1 tablespoon (0.5 oz)	14.3	77.2	1.4	0.0	0.00	0.1	0.00	0.01	1.3	3.0	0.00	4.3	142.1
19	**Mayonnaise**, regular, 1 salad dressing packet (2 oz)	55.0	394.2	6.5	32.5	0.00	4.2	0.32	0.14	6.5	9.9	0.28	18.7	312.6
178	**Meat loaf** made with beef, 1 medium slice (3.8 oz)	108.0	229.3	4.9	89.1	0.44	16.3	0.14	1.64	0.1	43.1	2.02	293.4	435.4
154	**Muffin**, English, toasted, 1 muffin (1.75 oz)	50.0	127.5	0.1	0.0	1.45	37.0	0.02	0.02	0.1	94.5	1.36	71.5	252.0
146	**Muffin**, fruit and/or nuts, 1 medium muffin (2-3/4", 2 oz)	57.0	157.9	0.8	17.1	1.48	25.7	0.01	0.33	0.6	32.5	0.92	70.1	254.8
15	**Mustard**, 1 packet (0.16 oz)	5.0	3.8	0.0	0.0	0.14	0.4	0.00	0.00	0.1	4.2	0.10	6.5	62.6
27	**Onion**, 1 medium (2-1/2", 3.9 oz)	110.0	41.8	0.0	0.0	1.98	20.9	0.13	0.00	0.1	22.0	0.24	172.7	3.3
43	**Orange**, 1 medium (2-5/8", 4.6 oz)	131.0	61.6	0.0	0.0	3.14	39.7	0.08	0.00	0.3	52.4	0.13	237.1	0.0
76	**Pancake**, plain, 1 medium pancake (5", 1.4 oz)	40.0	91.6	0.3	3.6	0.72	18.0	0.02	0.06	0.3	24.8	1.39	29.2	203.6
128	**Peach**, 1 medium (2-1/2", 3.5 oz)	98.0	42.1	0.0	0.0	1.96	3.3	0.02	0.00	0.7	4.9	0.11	193.1	0.0
35	**Peanut butter**, 1 tablespoon (0.6 oz)	16.0	94.9	1.7	0.0	0.94	11.8	0.07	0.00	1.6	6.1	0.29	107.0	74.7
163	**Pear**, 1 medium pear (5.9 oz)	166.0	97.9	0.0	0.0	3.98	12.1	0.03	0.00	0.8	18.3	0.42	207.5	0.0
132	**Pepper**, sweet, green, 1 medium (2-3/4" long, 2-1/2", 4.2 oz)	119.0	32.1	0.0	0.0	2.14	26.2	0.30	0.00	0.8	10.7	0.55	210.6	2.4
56	**Pickle**, dill, 1 medium (3-3/4" long, 2.3 oz)	65.0	11.7	0.0	0.0	0.78	0.7	0.01	0.00	0.1	5.9	0.34	75.4	833.3
111	**Pizza**, cheese, thin crust, 1 medium pizza (13", 20.8 oz)	590.0	1517.7	24.7	87.6	9.88	272.5	0.52	0.83	8.9	1378.1	12.23	1250.7	3857.5
194	**Pizza** with meat and vegetables, thin crust, 1 medium pizza (13", 26.1 oz)	740.0	1809.1	34.5	148.7	12.60	272.2	0.87	2.21	9.6	1268.4	13.98	1704.3	4768.4
131	**Pizza** with meat, thick crust, 1 medium pizza (13", 26.1 oz)	740.0	2280.1	35.0	134.8	12.31	410.9	0.62	2.01	9.8	1131.3	18.32	1404.9	5049.8
69	**Pizza** with meat, thin crust, 1 medium pizza (13", 23.5 oz)	666.0	1953.2	38.7	168.9	9.86	275.5	0.69	2.52	9.1	1384.6	13.73	1529.4	5106.0
141	**Popcorn**, popped in oil, buttered, 1 cup, popped (0.5 oz)	14.0	72.9	1.3	3.0	1.26	2.2	0.03	0.00	0.0	1.6	0.35	28.8	123.0
188	**Popcorn**, popped in oil, unbuttered, 1 cup, popped (0.4 oz)	11.0	55.0	0.5	0.0	1.10	1.9	0.02	0.00	0.0	1.1	0.31	24.8	97.2
46	**Pork bacon**, smoked or cured, 1 medium slice (0.3 oz cooked)	8.0	46.1	1.4	6.8	0.00	0.4	0.02	0.14	0.0	1.0	0.13	38.9	127.7
103	**Pork sausage**, 1 patty (3-7/8" dia x 1/4" thick raw, 1 oz cooked)	27.0	99.6	2.9	22.4	0.00	0.5	0.09	0.47	0.0	8.6	0.34	97.5	349.4
125	**Potato**, baked, peel eaten, 1 medium (2-1/4" to 3", 4.3 oz)	122.0	132.2	0.0	0.0	2.91	13.3	0.42	0.00	0.1	12.3	1.65	507.0	288.9
79	**Potato**, baked, peel not eaten, 1 medium (2-1/4" to 3")	98.0	90.6	0.0	0.0	1.46	8.9	0.29	0.00	0.1	5.0	0.34	380.9	237.2
198	**Potato**, oiled, without peel, 1 medium (2-1/4" to 3" dia, 4.3 oz)	122.0	104.3	0.0	0.0	2.18	10.8	0.33	0.00	0.1	9.9	0.38	397.8	295.3
25	**Potato**, chips, 1 chip, regular (0.05 oz)	1.4	7.5	0.2	0.0	0.06	0.6	0.01	0.00	0.1	0.3	0.02	17.9	8.3
20	**Potato**, french fries, 1 fast food order (3.5 oz)	100.0	309.1	5.0	0.4	3.20	33.0	0.26	0.12	0.2	16.0	1.35	712.0	163.0
68	**Potato**, french fries, 10 strips (2" to 3-1/2", 1.75 oz)	50.0	140.7	2.0	0.1	1.60	13.9	0.14	0.05	0.1	7.0	0.66	318.8	93.8
108	**Potato**, home fries, 1 medium potato (2-1/4" to 3", 2.5 oz)	70.0	96.8	0.6	0.0	1.17	6.4	0.18	0.00	1.0	4.5	0.20	228.7	162.5
73	**Potato**, mashed from fresh, made with milk and fat, 1 cup (7.4 oz)	210.0	225.8	1.8	2.4	3.07	16.7	0.47	0.11	1.2	51.8	0.55	608.7	658.8
180	**Potato salad**, 1 cup (6.8 oz)	193.0	274.8	2.3	11.0	3.10	21.5	0.55	0.05	2.4	21.0	0.79	594.2	799.6
64	**Pretzel**, hard, 1-3 ring pretzel (0.1 oz)	3.0	11.4	0.0	0.0	0.10	5.1	0.00	0.00	0.0	1.1	0.13	4.4	51.5
189	**Radish**, 1 medium (3/4" to 1", 0.15 oz)	4.5	0.9	0.0	0.0	0.07	1.2	0.00	0.00	0.0	0.9	0.01	10.4	1.1
190	**Raisins**, 50 raisins (0.9 oz)	26.0	78.0	0.0	0.0	1.04	0.9	0.06	0.00	0.2	12.7	0.54	195.3	3.1
164	**Refried beans**, 1 cup (8.9 oz)	253.0	484.8	8.8	20.7	17.57	323.1	0.37	0.00	2.1	108.8	5.23	993.1	665.5
173	**Rice Krispies**, 1 cup (0.9 oz)	26.0	98.0	0.1	0.0	0.29	91.8	0.44	0.00	0.0	2.6	1.56	33.3	278.7
92	**Rice**, white, fat added in cooking, 1 cup cooked (5.75 oz)	163.0	263.5	1.5	0.0	0.61	88.5	0.14	0.01	1.2	18.3	1.84	57.3	648.1
44	**Rice**, white, fat not added in cooking, 1 cup cooked (5.6 oz)	158.0	203.5	0.1	0.0	0.63	90.8	0.15	0.00	0.1	16.0	1.88	54.9	577.5
187	**Salami**, 1 slice (4" dia x 1/8" thick, 0.8 oz)	23.0	57.5	1.9	15.0	0.00	0.5	0.05	0.84	0.1	3.0	0.61	45.5	245.0
75	**Salsa**, red, cooked, not homemade, 1 tablespoon (0.5 fl oz)	16.0	3.5	0.0	0.0	0.30	2.2	0.02	0.00	0.1	7.4	0.12	29.6	41.4
155	**Soup**, mostly noodles, 1 cup (8 fl oz)	233.0	157.6	1.7	0.2	1.19	3.2	0.01	0.00	2.4	13.4	0.40	50.4	823.1
121	**Sour cream**, 1 cup (8 fl oz)	230.0	492.8	30.0	102.1	0.00	24.8	0.04	0.69	1.3	267.7	0.14	331.2	122.6
193	**Soy sauce**, 1 tablespoon (0.5 fl oz)	16.0	8.5	0.0	0.0	0.13	2.5	0.03	0.00	0.0	2.7	0.32	28.8	914.4
93	**Spaghetti**, plain, fat not added in cooking, 1 cup, cooked (4.9 oz)	140.0	196.2	0.1	0.0	2.37	97.4	0.05	0.00	0.1	9.9	1.95	43.2	325.0
140	**Spaghetti** with tomato sauce and meatballs or meat sauce, 1 cup (8.8 oz)	248.0	323.4	3.2	68.3	3.64	76.0	0.35	1.01	2.1	129.6	3.72	650.4	1075.8
113	**Spaghetti sauce**, 1 cup (8.8 oz)	250.0	142.5	0.7	0.0	4.00	25.0	0.29	0.00	3.1	55.0	1.80	737.5	1030.0
142	**Spaghetti sauce** with beef, homemade-style, 1 cup (8.8 oz)	249.0	287.7	4.5	46.6	4.20	29.8	0.54	1.44	5.3	59.0	3.53	1100.0	1177.4
89	**Strawberries**, 1 cup, whole (5.1 oz)	144.0	43.2	0.0	0.0	3.31	25.5	0.08	0.00	0.2	20.2	0.55	239.0	1.4
58	**Sugar substitute**, aspartame-based, dry powder, 1 individual packet	1.0	3.5	0.0	0.0	0.00	0.0	0.00	0.00	0.0	0.0	0.00	0.0	0.0

Rank		Grams	Calories	Sat Fat	Cholesterol	Fiber	Folate	Vitamin B6	Vitamin B12	Vitamin E	Calcium	Iron	Potassium	Sodium
		g	kcal	g	mg	g	mg	mg	mcg	ATE	mg	mg	mg	mg
36	**Sugar substitute,** saccharin-based, dry powder, 1 individual packet	1.0	3.6	0.0	0.0	0.00	0.0	0.00	0.00	0.0	0.0	0.00	45.0	4.0
5	**Sugar,** white, granulated or lump, 1 teaspoon (0.15 oz)	4.2	16.3	0.0	0.0	0.00	0.0	0.00	0.00	0.0	0.0	0.00	0.1	0.0
156	**Tart,** breakfast, 1 Pop Tart (1.8 oz)	52.0	204.4	0.8	0.0	1.09	33.8	0.20	0.03	1.0	13.5	1.81	58.2	217.9
7	**Tomato,** raw, 1 medium whole (2-3/5", 4.3 oz)	123.0	25.8	0.1	0.0	1.35	18.5	0.10	0.00	0.5	6.2	0.55	273.1	11.1
11	**Tomato catsup,** 1 tablespoon (0.5 oz)	15.0	15.6	0.0	0.0	0.20	2.3	0.03	0.00	0.2	2.9	0.11	72.2	177.9
45	**Tortilla chips,** 10 chips (0.6 oz)	18.0	90.2	0.9	0.0	1.17	1.8	0.05	0.00	0.2	27.7	0.27	35.5	95.0
97	**Tortilla, corn,** 1 medium tortilla (approx 6", 0.7 oz)	19.0	42.2	0.1	0.0	0.99	21.7	0.04	0.00	0.0	33.3	0.27	29.3	30.6
133	**Tuna salad,** 1 cup (7.3 oz)	208.0	295.6	1.7	41.4	0.96	14.7	0.44	3.43	1.9	27.5	2.15	351.9	853.5
119	**Waffle,** plain, 1 square waffle (4" square, 1.3 oz)	37.0	97.7	0.5	8.9	0.85	16.7	0.33	0.93	0.3	85.8	1.65	47.4	291.2
109	**Water** as an ingredient, 1 cup (8 fl oz)	237.0	0.0	0.0	0.0	0.00	0.0	0.00	0.00	0.0	4.7	0.02	0.0	7.1
98	**Watermelon,** 1 wedge (1/16 of melon, 10 oz)	286.0	91.5	0.1	0.0	1.43	6.3	0.41	0.00	0.4	22.9	0.49	331.8	5.7

Drinks

Rank		Grams	Calories	Sat Fat	Cholesterol	Fiber	Folate	Vitamin B6	Vitamin B12	Vitamin E	Calcium	Iron	Potassium	Sodium
72	**Apple juice,** 1 cup (8 fl oz)	248.0	116.6	0.0	0.0	0.25	0.2	0.07	0.00	0.0	17.4	0.92	295.1	7.4
40	**Beer,** 1 can or bottle (12 fl oz)	360.0	147.6	0.0	0.0	0.72	21.6	0.18	0.07	0.0	18.0	0.11	90.0	18.0
71	**Beer, lite,** 1 can or bottle (12 fl oz)	360.0	100.8	0.0	0.0	0.00	14.8	0.12	0.04	0.0	18.0	0.14	64.8	10.8
34	**Coffee,** regular, from powdered instant, 1 coffee cup (6 fl oz)	179.0	3.9	0.0	0.0	0.00	0.0	0.00	0.00	0.0	5.8	0.09	57.7	5.9
1	**Coffee,** regular, ground, 1 coffee cup (6 fl oz)	177.0	3.5	0.0	0.0	0.00	0.2	0.00	0.00	0.0	3.5	0.09	95.6	3.5
81	**Coffee,** decaffeinated, from powdered instant, 1 coffee cup (6 fl oz)	179.0	3.7	0.0	0.0	0.00	0.0	0.00	0.00	0.0	5.8	0.08	57.2	5.7
41	**Coffee,** decaffeinated, ground, 1 coffee cup (6 fl oz)	177.0	3.5	0.0	0.0	0.00	0.0	0.00	0.00	0.0	3.5	0.09	95.6	3.5
2	**Cola-type soft drink,** 1 can (12 fl oz)	369.0	151.3	0.0	0.0	0.00	0.0	0.00	0.00	0.0	11.1	0.11	3.7	14.8
137	**Cola-type soft drink,** decaffeinated, 1 can (12 fl oz)	369.0	151.3	0.0	0.0	0.00	0.0	0.00	0.00	0.0	11.1	0.11	3.7	14.8
61	**Cola-type soft drink,** decaffeinated, sugar-free, 1 can (12 fl oz)	355.0	3.6	0.0	0.0	0.00	0.0	0.00	0.00	0.0	14.2	0.11	0.0	21.3
16	**Cola-type soft drink,** sugar-free, 1 can (12 fl oz)	355.0	3.6	0.0	0.0	0.00	0.0	0.00	0.00	0.0	14.2	0.11	0.0	21.3
151	**Cranberry juice** drink with vitamin C added, 1 cup (8 fl oz)	253.0	144.2	0.0	0.0	0.25	0.5	0.05	0.00	0.0	7.6	0.38	45.5	5.1
78	**Fruit drink,** 1 cup (8 fl oz)	248.0	116.6	0.0	0.0	0.25	2.5	0.00	0.00	0.0	19.8	0.52	62.0	54.6
105	**Fruit punch,** fruit drink, or fruitade, with vitamin C added, 1 cup (8 fl oz)	247.0	116.1	0.0	0.0	0.25	3.2	0.00	0.00	0.0	19.8	0.52	61.8	54.3
101	**Fruit-flavored drink,** from sweetened powdered mix, 1 cup (8 fl oz)	250.0	87.8	0.0	0.0	0.02	0.2	0.00	0.00	0.0	37.2	0.14	1.2	34.4
67	**Fruit-flavored drink,** from unsweetened powdered mix, 1 cup (8 fl oz)	240.0	89.7	0.0	0.0	0.00	0.0	0.00	0.00	0.0	14.1	0.04	0.5	12.5
22	**Fruit-flavored soft drink,** caffeine free, 1 can (12 fl oz)	368.0	147.2	0.0	0.0	0.00	0.0	0.00	0.00	0.0	7.4	0.26	3.7	40.5
49	**Fruit-flavored soft drink,** containing caffeine, 1 can (12 fl oz)	372.0	148.8	0.0	0.0	0.00	0.0	0.00	0.00	0.0	7.4	0.26	3.7	40.9
143	**Fruit-flavored soft drink,** sugar free, caffeine free, 1 can (12 fl oz)	355.0	0.0	0.0	0.0	0.00	0.0	0.00	0.00	0.0	14.2	0.14	7.1	21.3
172	**Fruit-flavored thirst quencher** beverage, 1 cup (8 fl oz)	240.0	60.0	0.0	0.0	0.00	0.0	0.00	0.00	0.0	0.0	0.12	26.4	96.0
118	**Lemonade,** 1 Snapple bottle (16 fl oz)	496.0	198.7	0.0	0.0	0.44	11.0	0.03	0.00	0.0	15.4	0.83	73.6	16.0
18	**Milk,** 1% fat, 1 cup (8 fl oz)	244.0	102.1	1.6	9.8	0.00	12.4	0.10	0.90	0.1	300.1	0.12	380.9	123.2
3	**Milk,** 2% fat, 1 cup (8 fl oz)	244.0	121.2	2.9	18.3	0.00	12.4	0.10	0.89	0.2	296.7	0.12	376.7	121.8
10	**Milk,** skim or nonfat, 0.5% or less butterfat, 1 cup (8 fl oz)	245.0	85.5	0.3	4.4	0.00	12.7	0.10	0.93	0.1	302.3	0.10	405.7	126.2
4	**Milk,** whole, 1 cup (8 fl oz)	244.0	149.9	5.1	33.2	0.00	12.2	0.10	0.87	0.2	291.3	0.12	369.7	119.6
149	**Milk,** chocolate, reduced fat, 1 cup (8 fl oz)	250.0	178.8	3.1	17.0	1.25	12.0	0.10	0.85	0.1	284.0	0.60	422.0	150.5
127	**Orange breakfast drink,** 1 cup (8 fl oz)	250.0	110.0	0.0	0.0	0.00	20.0	0.03	0.00	0.0	10.0	0.10	102.5	160.0
13	**Orange juice,** unsweetened, 1 cup (8 fl oz)	249.0	104.6	0.0	0.0	0.50	45.1	0.22	0.00	0.2	19.9	1.10	435.8	5.0
42	**Orange juice,** frozen, unsweetened (with water), 1 cup (8 fl oz)	249.0	113.0	0.0	0.0	0.57	110.4	0.11	0.00	0.2	26.3	0.27	479.0	7.5
134	**Root beer,** 1 can (12 fl oz)	370.0	151.7	0.0	0.0	0.00	0.0	0.00	0.00	0.0	18.5	0.19	3.7	48.1
50	**Soft drink, pepper-type,** 1 can (12 fl oz)	369.0	151.3	0.0	0.0	0.00	0.0	0.00	0.00	0.0	11.1	0.11	3.7	14.8
153	**Tea,** herbal, 1 teacup (6 fl oz)	178.0	1.8	0.0	0.0	0.00	1.1	0.00	0.00	0.0	3.6	0.14	16.0	1.8
148	**Tea,** leaf, decaffeinated, unsweetened, 1 teacup (6 fl oz)	178.0	1.8	0.0	0.0	0.00	8.9	0.00	0.00	0.0	0.0	0.04	65.9	5.3
39	**Tea,** leaf, presweetened, 1 fl oz	29.6	6.0	0.0	0.0	0.00	1.5	0.00	0.00	0.0	0.0	0.01	10.4	0.9
14	**Tea,** leaf, unsweetened, 1 teacup (6 fl oz)	178.0	1.8	0.0	0.0	0.00	9.3	0.00	0.00	0.0	0.0	0.04	65.9	5.3
166	**Tea,** made from powdered instant, presweetened, 1 teacup (6 fl oz)	178.0	17.5	0.0	0.0	0.02	0.7	0.01	0.00	0.0	3.9	0.05	45.1	6.1
74	**Wine,** table, dry, 1 wine glass (3.5 fl oz)	103.0	72.1	0.0	0.0	0.00	1.1	0.02	0.01	0.0	8.2	0.42	91.7	8.2

Food measurements:
1 ounce (oz) = 28.35 grams (g)
1 fluid ounce (fl oz) = 29.6 milliliters (ml)
1 pound = 16 oz (453.6g)

1 tablespoon = 3 teaspoons = 1/2 fl oz (14.8 ml)
1 cup = 8 fl oz (236.6 ml)
1 pint = 16 fl oz (473.2 ml)

1 kg (1000g) = 35.3 oz
1 liter (1000 ml) = 33.8 fl oz

About Stikky books

The Stikky story

We started publishing Stikky books in 2003 after a web-based trial generated far more interest than we expected. Our first book, *Stikky Night Skies*, took a year to create.

The series covers topics we believe will be of value and interest to anyone. We created it because we couldn't find a 'how to' book that took into account recent findings about how people learn. Instead, they often provide too much information and structure it in a way that makes sense to experts but not to beginners. According to our research, most people read less than half of 'how to' books they buy.

The Stikky approach

- Start with small pieces of knowledge and systematically build them into a comprehensive picture
- Make the practice environment as similar as possible to the real world
- Organize the topic around readers' goals such as: How do I read a nutrition label?
- Provide plenty of practice—80% of learning is really re-learning so we stage multiple opportunities to test and reinforce your knowledge
- Make it fun.

How we create a Stikky book

Each book is prepared with the help of subject experts, some of whom are named on the cover. It goes through multiple rounds of review by Test Readers. (If you would like to become a Stikky Test Reader, visit www.stikky.com). We record every time they get stuck, together with hundreds of other suggestions, and make careful changes. Then we go through the whole process again.

Everything about the product in your hands was informed by this research: the format, the binding, even the name. And we only publish a book when we know it works.

Our charity pledge

We promise to spend 10% of profits from the series on knowledge-based charity. We believe that knowledge generates independence and so is a liberating form of aid.

Upcoming Stikky books

Future titles will cover topics such as the secrets of persuasion or playing a musical instrument. If there are topics you would like to see included in the series, suggest them at www.stikky.com, where you will also find news of additions to the series before their publication.

What our readers say

Comments from readers of Stikky books

15 minutes with this book was more valuable than the 3 hours I spent stumbling with another. *BM, USA*

Amazing…so simple and so thorough. *MW, UK*

After running through the sequence, I was able to locate all the points very quickly, can't wait to try it out. *PP, Australia*

Within 30 minutes this book has provided a basis for me to begin a new adventure and hobby. *BR, Indiana*

Yes, my brain is full, and I don't have time to learn anything new. But the folks who created this book are on to something. *A reader from Palo Alto, California*

If you've ever had a teacher who explained things in such a way that they stikk to your mind forever, this book will let you re-live that experience. *SN, New Jersey*

I felt successful from the start. *JC, UK*

This book at first seemed too simple. Then after buying and reading it, I realized it was perfect. The information is presented in such a way that I feel I'll retain the knowledge for life. *A reader from Dallas, Texas*

I have read many, many books on constellations, but this is the most effective one I have ever seen. *WR, Canada*

Now I can observe and understand with confidence. Thank you so much. *LC, Michigan*

Thank you so much for making things so easy. I feel like I've made a start, at long last. *CW, England*

We need more teachers/educators with this approach. *JF, USA*

What a magnificent idea! I will email everybody I know that even MIGHT be interested! Please PLEASE create more of these. *DJ, Ohio*

Beautifully simple, entertaining and delightful. *PL, Ontario*

Thank You

Quentin Ball · Jonathan Bloom · Annette Brookman · Victoria Cable-Kulli · Merry Davis · Alberta Eng
Jessica Fracassini · Colleen Helmken · Andrew Lyons · Miranda McGrath · Rafael Mestre · John Oakes
Damien Offord · Mark Rossetti · Earle Sandberg · Maureen Shannon · Clare Smith · Leah Soufrant